The Juice Lady's™

Juicing for High-Level Wellness and Vibrant Good Looks

ALSO BY CHERIE CALBOM

Juicing for Life
with Maureen Keane

———————————

The Healthy Gourmet

———————————

*Knock-Out-the-Fat Barbecue
and Grilling Cookbook*
with George Foreman

The Juice Lady's™
Juicing for High-Level Wellness and Vibrant Good Looks

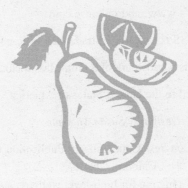

by Cherie Calbom, M.S.

Three Rivers Press
New York

Published by Three Rivers Press, 201 East 50th Street, New York, New York 10022. Member of the Crown Publishing Group.

Random House, Inc. New York, Toronto, London, Sydney, Auckland

www.randomhouse.com

THREE RIVERS PRESS is a registered trademark of Random House, Inc.

THE JUICE LADY is a trademark of Salton-Maxim Housewares, Inc.

Printed in the United States of America

Design by Susan Maksuta

Library of Congress Cataloging-in-Publication Data
Calbom, Cherie.
The juice lady™'s juicing for high-level wellness and vibrant good looks / by Cherie Calbom. — 1st pbk. ed.
Includes index.
1. Fruit juices—Health aspects.   2. Vegetable juices—Health aspects.   I. Title.
RA784.C229   1998
613.2'6—dc21
98-35517
CIP

ISBN 0-609-80349-2

10 9 8 7 6 5 4 3 2

To my grandmother, Minnie Neely Batdorf,
who grew a bountiful organic garden year after year
and was my first teacher of natural medicine.

Acknowledgments

I wish to express my deep and lasting appreciation to the people who have assisted me with this book, especially Joanna Burgess for her creative writing assistance.

A heartfelt thanks to the Nutrition Department of Bastyr University, especially Dr. Mark Kestin and Alia Calendar, whose help was invaluable in coordinating the research for my book. A special thanks to the following Bastyr University students who did a superb job researching various topics for "Juicing for High-Level Wellness": Catherine Mourey, Artemis Morris, Terry Monaghan, Pushpa Larsen-Giacalone, Carolyn Bell, Trina Fykerud, Kelly Morrow, Nicole Jensen, Beth DiDomenico, Norlinda Ghazali, Patti Pritchard, and Laura Behenna.

A very special thanks to Wendy Keller, my agent, for her expert help and guidance.

Much thanks to my editor, Peter Guzzardi, for working overtime to make this project a success.

Finally, deep gratitude and continued appreciation to John, my husband and "official taste tester," who drank juice and smoothies until he couldn't take another sip.

Contents

The Juice Lady's™

Juicing for High-Level Wellness and Vibrant Good Looks

Introduction

People often ask me how I became the "Juice Lady." If they've never tried juicing before, they wonder why I'm so excited about fresh juice. Occasionally, some think I'm a full-fledged health nut. This reaction continues to amaze me. Our culture teaches us that processed foods, filled with preservatives and synthetic additives, are somehow "natural" and much better for us than fruits and vegetables! Doesn't it just make sense that produce from backyard gardens or organic farms is healthier than boxed food from a factory with a shelf life of ten years?

When I tell people the truth behind my conversion, their jaws drop with surprise. I became interested in juicing out of desperation. Never having considered the connection between a healthy diet and a healthy body, I rarely thought twice about what I put into my body. Though I lived with my maternal grandmother, who grew a bountiful organic garden each year and prepared lots of vegetables at meals, I didn't think most of them were particularly appealing. I liked eating sweet peas and baby carrots right out of the garden and corn on the cob with lots of butter, but that was about it. For the most part, my diet centered around my grandmother's homemade bread with plenty of butter and generous amounts of sweets. I loved junk food and didn't get nearly enough exercise.

Throughout grade school and junior high, I caught nearly every cold and flu bug that circulated in school and was often sidelined due to my low energy level and susceptibility to illness. There were many mornings I found myself so exhausted that I was barely able to crawl out of bed. My childhood doctors attributed my fragile health to family history—my mother died of cancer when I was six years old—and were at a loss to help. Feeling unwell and tired became a natural state of being for me, one I accepted without much thought for many years.

My health continued to fluctuate throughout my teens and twenties. In order to stay thin, I'd put myself on crash or starvation diets. An aunt convinced me to take vitamin and mineral pills. While my energy would noticeably increase while I was taking them, I still suffered bouts of fatigue and recurring illnesses. Whatever good I was doing taking my vitamins was almost canceled out by my poor diet and the large quantities of sugar I was

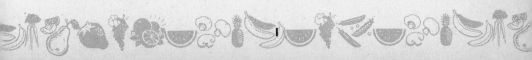

still consuming. I hated the thought of eating vegetables—to me they seemed to take too much time to prepare and were boring.

The crisis came when I turned thirty and developed a full-blown case of chronic fatigue syndrome. I was perennially lethargic, and I felt as if I had a continual case of the flu. My body was in constant pain and I was also suffering from what is now known as fibromyalgia. Within a few months, I had developed an acute ache in my lower back and was diagnosed with hypoglycemia and *Candida albicans* (a systemic yeast infection). I had never felt worse, and my situation was quickly becoming desperate. I visited a holistic doctor, who tested me for hundreds of allergies. When he finished, I walked out of his office with a list of food allergies longer than my arm and felt more discouraged and lost than ever.

I got so sick that I was forced to quit my job and move back to my father's house. Being someone who doesn't like to give up, I decided to find an answer to my health problems on my own. I couldn't afford to spend the next few months in bed, and I needed to find an effective, reliable, and affordable solution as quickly as possible. I began visiting a local health food store and talking to the employees there to see if they had any suggestions. I also read any health-related material that I could get my hands on. Finally I stumbled across a book about juicing by Norman Walker. With nothing to lose but my ill health, I decided to give juicing a try—it's a decision that saved my life and changed my outlook on food forever.

I began a five-day juice fast, focusing almost entirely on vegetable juices. I learned that my body responds negatively to sugar, so for me it was best to keep fruit juices, which contain sugar naturally, to a minimum. During my fast, I ate nothing solid and eliminated toxins from my body by using a cleansing program. For the rest of the summer, I followed a detoxification program. I eliminated all processed foods from my diet, drastically cut my intake of meat and poultry, drank four to six glasses of fresh, organic vegetable juice each day, and did periodic juice fasts to keep my system healthy and strong. The results were truly astounding. By September, just three months after starting my fresh juice program, my symptoms had virtually disappeared. My pain and fatigue were gone, and so were most of my food allergies. I had to follow an anti-*Candida* program to get rid of my yeast condition, but it eventually cleared up as well. I felt healthy, strong, and fit—three adjectives I had never before used in describing myself.

Juicing changed my emotional and intellectual relationship with food as well. I decided that I wanted to devote my life to the pursuit of health. I went to a career development class and, with the help of a very supportive teacher (my husband!), discovered that a career as a nutritionist was the perfect outlet for me to pursue my dream. While getting my master's in nutrition at Bastyr University in Seattle, Washington, I got a job writing a booklet on juice for the Juiceman Juicer. After finishing the booklet, the company that produced the Juiceman Juicer asked me to teach national seminars about juicing. It was the perfect opportunity to interact with people and learn about different health needs while teaching vital nutritional facts about the benefits of juicing and eating healthy. I began traveling across the country and conducting seminars on the benefits of juicing. I continually spoke to rooms full of people suffering from ailments that conventional medicine couldn't fix. It made me realize just how many people out there are looking for natural solutions to disorders, and I was very glad that I had a reliable alternative to offer them.

My hectic schedule took its toll on my body, however. In 1993, after almost two years on the road, I began to get sick again. I had been traveling so much teaching people how to use juicing to promote their own health that I had begun to neglect my own. My chronic fatigue syndrome and fibromyalgia returned. Moving to a new city every few days didn't exactly afford me the time to juice for myself or exercise properly. I often relied on fruit juice prepared on stage during my seminars, along with restaurant food, to get me through a day of lectures. I decided to take some time off, get back on my vegetable juicing program, and restore my body to health. By the end of 1993, I was well again. In 1994, I wrote *The Healthy Gourmet,* a cookbook dedicated to simple, nutritious, and tasty meals. After finishing my book, I attended a trade show sponsored by the makers of the Juiceman Juicer, Salton-Maxim Housewares, where I met boxer George Foreman, who was promoting his Lean Mean Fat-Reducing Grilling Machine. He was so delighted by the benefits of juicing and my recipes that he asked me to be his personal nutritionist. In 1995, I wrote *Knock-Out-the-Fat Barbecue and Grilling Cookbook* with George and began appearing with him at trade shows and on TV.

The CEO at Salton-Maxim was impressed by my scientific understanding and approach to juicing and asked me to develop my own line of juicers. Thus, the Juice Lady™ Pro Series was born. I've been selling the Juice Lady™ 210 on The Shopping Channel of Canada (TSC) and QVC for the past two years and launched the Juice Lady™ Pro, The Next Generation of juicers in 1999.

I think what people most often realize after they start juicing is that it's the easiest, most convenient way of making vegetable and fruit consumption a habit. They're amazed at how simple it is to take control of their health and begin feeling more energetic and more alive. Fresh juices are packed with vitamins, minerals, enzymes, and phytonutrients, so there's no more worrying about meeting the recommended daily allowance (RDA) of fruits and vegetables with every meal. They also contain a special energy from the sun made available to us through photosynthesis. Two or three glasses of fresh, organic veggie or fruit juice is all it takes to get an abundance of life-giving nutrients. And most parents are pleasantly surprised to discover that their kids will gladly swap soda pop for homemade fruit smoothies and fresh fruit and vegetable juices.

My personal experiences, and those of my friends, family, associates, and people I've met throughout the years, convince me that juicing is a natural way to revitalize the body and the cornerstone of staying fit, healthy, and young. If I had never taken the initiative and searched out a natural healing practice, I know I would have spent the rest of my life suffering from illness, chronic pain, and lasting fatigue. And worse, I may have developed a life-threatening disease. Juicing has enabled me to heal my body, take control of my health, and share with thousands of people around the world the essence of nature and the building blocks of life.

I wish you the best of success with your juicing. Here's to your health!

Why Juice?

If we ate the recommended five to nine servings of fruits and vegetables every day, we would be much closer to getting the nutrients we need to prevent disease and experience good health. Sadly, surveys show that less than 9 percent of the U.S. population eats even the minimum of two or more servings of fruit and three or more servings of vegetables per day. The Second National Health and Nutrition Examination found that a one-day look at the diet of 12,000 Americans showed that 41 percent ate no fruit on that survey day and only 25 percent reported eating one fruit or vegetable rich in beta carotene or vitamin C.

Most Americans are missing important vitamins, minerals, enzymes, and the newly discovered *phytochemicals,* also known as *phytonutrients* (*phyto* means plant), because they don't eat enough fruits and vegetables. Scientists believe phytochemicals may prove to be even more important than vitamins and minerals in keeping us healthy. Without an ample amount of all the nutrients found primarily in plants, the immune system weakens, we feel fatigued, and ailments and diseases develop.

Did you ever think about the fact that every time you eat a fruit or a vegetable, you are juicing it? Your teeth are grinding up a sweet peach or crunching into a crisp carrot and separating the juice from the fiber. That takes a lot of time. I timed eating a medium-size carrot one day to see how long it would take. Ten minutes. I don't have 50 to 60 minutes on most days of the week to spend eating 5 to 6 carrots. How about you? But I do eat that many carrots almost every day because I juice them; therefore, I'm getting an abundance of beta carotene and other carotenoids, along with a host of additional nutrients from the carrots, beets, celery, parsley, ginger, lemon, and spinach that my husband and I juice in the morning and from the tomato, cucumber, fennel, and lemon we juice in the afternoon. Therefore, I always advise that people eat fruits and vegetables whenever possible and drink juices, especially vegetable juices, every day.

Four Reasons to Juice Your Own Produce and to Juice Every Day

1. *Juicing is fast.*   Fresh juice is the healthiest fast food on earth, I say. It provides a quick, easy way to eat some of your five to nine servings of fruits and vegetables each day.

2. *Juice is rich in antioxidants.*   In the past, naysayers have purported that many of the precious vitamins and minerals in fruits and vegetables were actually trapped in the fiber and were not available in the juice. But in 1996 the U.S. Department of Agriculture conducted a study that disproved that theory completely. Twelve fruits were analyzed, and it was found that 90 percent of the antioxidant activity—that's beta carotene (provitamin A), vitamins C and E, and selenium—was in the juice rather than in the fiber. Eat fiber-rich fruits and vegetables, and juice even more of them to get an abundance of the antioxidants from the juice.

3. *Juice provides an abundance of enzymes, vitamins, minerals, and phytochemicals.*   Cooking, even steaming, vegetables destroys many of the enzymes and vitamins your body needs to stay healthy. The National Food Review Board says that cooking and freezing can destroy a large percentage of the nutrients in many foods.

Fresh juice isn't just another beverage that tastes good; it is a vitamin-mineral-rich cocktail in a glass. Freshly made juice is far superior to canned, bottled, or frozen juice because the vitamins, phytochemicals, and enzymes have not been destroyed by pasteurization. Pasteurization is the process of sterilization of a fluid at high temperatures to destroy objectionable organisms. Unfortunately, pasteurizing juice also destroys the fragile nutrients we want most because they can't withstand high heat.

4. *You can choose organic fruits and vegetables and the best produce.* When you make your own juice, you can choose organic produce (see Organically Grown, page 180) and thereby avoid pesticides, herbicides, and chemical fertilizers. In addition, you can select the choicest fruits and vegetables. With commercial juice, you never know the condition of the fruits and vegetables chosen for making juice. Were they bruised, moldy, or damaged? Did they come from another country where chemicals such as DDT (banned in this country) may have been used? Were they irradiated, a very frightening practice regarding our health?

TIPS FOR JUICING

1. Wash all produce before juicing; fruit and vegetable washes are available from many grocers and health food stores. Cut away all moldy, bruised, or damaged areas before juicing.

2. Use organic or unsprayed (transitional) produce whenever possible to ensure that you have the purest juices possible. (See Organically Grown, page 180.)

3. Because the skins of oranges, tangerines, and grapefruits contain indigestible, volatile oils that can cause digestive problems and taste bitter, always peel these citrus fruits before juicing. (Lemon and lime peels can be juiced, if organic.) You should leave as much of the white pithy part on the citrus fruit as possible, since it contains the most vitamin C and bioflavonoids (phytonutrients with antioxidant activity). Always peel mangos and papayas, since their skins contain an irritant that is harmful when eaten in quantity. Also, I recommend that you peel all produce that is not labeled organic, even though the largest concentration of nutrients is in and next to the skin; the peels and skins of sprayed fruits and vegetables have the largest concentration of pesticides.

4. Remove pits, stones, and hard seeds from fruits such as peaches, plums, apricots, cherries, and mangos. Softer seeds from oranges, lemons, watermelon, cantaloupe, grapes, and apples can be juiced without a problem. Because of their chemical composition, large quantities of apple seeds should not be juiced for young children; they should be okay for adults.

5. The stems and leaves of most produce, such as beet stems and leaves, strawberry caps, and small grape stems, can be included in the juicing process; they offer nutrients as well. Larger grape stems should be discarded as they can dull the juicer blade. Carrot and rhubarb greens should be removed, however, because they contain toxic substances.

6. Most fruits and vegetables have a high water content, which makes them ideal for juicing. Those with much less water, such as banana, mango, papaya, and avocado, will not juice well. They can be used in smoothies and cold soups by combining them with fresh juice in a blender (for recipes, see pages 13–67).

7. Most fruits and vegetables should be cut into sections or pieces that will fit your juicer's feed tube.

8. Juice can be stored in an airtight, opaque container in the refrigerator or in a thermos for up to 24 hours; light, heat, and air will destroy nutrients quickly. Melon and cabbage juices do not store well. Be aware that the longer juice sits before you drink it, the more nutrients it loses. If juice turns brown, it has oxidized and lost a large amount of its food value. After 24 hours, it may spoil.

9. Place a thin plastic bag—the kind that is free in the produce section of a grocery store—in the pulp receptacle of your juicer. When you are done juicing, you can toss the pulp or use it in cooking or composting, but you won't need to wash the receptacle.

LOOK WHAT'S IN FRESH JUICE!

Carbohydrates are formed when carbon dioxide and water come together in the presence of sunlight and chlorophyll (the green pigment in plants). The chemical bonds of the carbohydrate lock in the energy of the sun, and this energy is released when the body burns plant food as fuel. There are three types of carbohydrates: simple (sugars), complex (starches), and fiber. Soluble fiber is found in juice, and insoluble fiber is found in whole fruits, vegetables, whole grains, and legumes.

Protein is the most plentiful substance in the body, after water. Fresh juice contains amino acids and small amounts of protein. Combine with legumes (beans, lentils, split peas) and whole grains to boost protein levels if you are a vegetarian.

Fats in the form of essential fatty acids are available in vegetables, seeds, and nuts. These are the "good fats" that reduce your risk of heart disease and other diseases and that make your skin soft and your hair shiny.

Vitamins are needed by the body for normal growth and tissue maintenance. Even though they are needed in only small amounts, most vitamins must be supplied through your diet because the body cannot manufacture them. They are divided into two groups: water-soluble vitamins that include the B-complex vitamins and vitamin C, and fat-soluble vitamins that include vitamins A, D, E, and K. The body can store fat-soluble vitamins,

CHOOSING THE RIGHT JUICER

Choosing the right juicer can make the difference between juicing often and never juicing again. Of course, I recommend the Juice Lady brand; indeed, the Juice Lady is the best machine I have used. But whether you choose one of my machines or not, look for the following features:

1. A quality motor is essential. Choose one with a .5-horsepower motor if you want it to last a long time. Smaller motors can burn out quickly or work so poorly that juicing is more effort than it is worth. The Juice Lady 210 juicer has a .25-horsepower motor and will not last as long, but is a good machine at an affordable price. It will juice everything the larger machines can process.

2. Choose a juicer with only a few parts to clean. The more parts you have to wash, the longer it will take you to clean the juicer and put it back together. Cleaning time for three or four parts should be just a couple of minutes.

3. A juicer that ejects pulp into a receptacle is far better than one that keeps all the pulp inside where it has to be scooped out continually. A juicer that keeps the pulp in the center basket rather than ejecting it cannot do continuous juicing; you'll need to stop often and wash it out. High-powered, blender-type juicers that keep all the pulp in the juice do not produce a delicious-tasting juice. Vegetable and herb pulp in juice is especially grainy and gritty.

4. Make sure the juicer can handle herbs and leafy greens—many cannot—and make sure that it does not require a special citrus attachment.

but water-soluble vitamins must be continually replenished. Fruit and vegetable juices are excellent sources of most of these vitamins.

Minerals are elements in their simple inorganic form. In the body, minerals occur primarily in the ionic form; metals form positive ions and nonmetals form negative ions. Minerals are used by the body in three major ways: to build structural tissues, such as calcium and magnesium, for bone; they are used in electrolyte balance, as is the case with potassium, sodium, chloride, and calcium; they also serve a function in metabolism, as is the case with zinc. The major minerals are calcium, chloride, magnesium, phosphorus, potassium, sodium, and sulfur. Trace minerals are those needed in very small amounts and include arsenic, boron, chromium, cobalt, copper, fluoride, manganese, nickel, selenium, vanadium, and zinc. Fruits and vegetables and their juices are among the best sources of minerals.

Enzymes are molecules that speed up chemical reactions necessary for human bodily functions. Enzymes are abundant in fresh fruits and vegetables and raw juices that have not been pasteurized. Enzymes work with coenzymes to either join molecules together or split them apart. An important concept in nutritional medicine is knowing how to supply the nutrients necessary to allow enzymes of a particular tissue to work at optimum level. Fresh juices package enzymes with vitamins, minerals, and phytonutrients, making available a wide spectrum of nutrients so that the enzymes can perform their functions. When a diet is low in raw fruits and vegetables, various organs and glands work overtime to provide enzymes for digestion and metabolism. Fresh juices, with their abundance of enzymes, can relieve those organs and glands from overwork.

Phytochemicals (natural plant nutrients) are tiny elements in plants that protect them from disease, injury, and pollution. Phytochemicals form the plant's first line of defense against disease. The good news is that they also help our own "superfighter" immune cells by strengthening and supporting the immune system. The National Cancer Institute has launched a multimillion-dollar project to find, isolate, and study cancer-preventing powers of phytochemicals.

Tens of thousands of phytochemicals have been discovered in recent years. Over the last 20 years, researchers have found that people who eat the most fruits and vegetables (the best sources of phytochemicals) have the lowest rates of cancers and other diseases. Following is a list of several of these plant heroes and what they do for us:

Lycopene, abundant in tomatoes, deters tumor growth and prostate disease.
Limonene, found in citrus fruits, stimulates enzymes that break down carcinogens.
Dithiolthiones, dominant in broccoli, helps in the formation of enzymes that may block carcinogens from damaging a cell's DNA.
Ellagic acid, found in grapes and strawberries, scavenges carcinogens and prevents them from altering the cells of DNA.

Caffeic acid, found in fruit, enhances the production of enzymes that make carcinogens more water soluble.

Indoles, found in cruciferous vegetables such as broccoli, cabbage, and cauliflower, stimulate enzymes that make the hormone estrogen less detrimental.

Chlorophyll, which gives green plants their color, detoxifies poisonous substances that can cause growths. It also improves skin texture and helps heal ulcers.

Gingerol, found in ginger root, reduces inflammation, helps lower cholesterol, and heals ulcers.

Just like the human body, fruits and vegetables are composed of a large percentage of *water.* Although we know we should drink eight to ten 8-ounce glasses of water per day to maintain good health, most of us don't. B. F. Batmanghelidj, M.D., says in his book, *Your Body's Many Cries for Water,* that you may not be sick, just thirsty. He explains that conditions such as rheumatoid arthritis may be caused by dehydrated joints. Low back pain may be due to a dehydrated disc core because 75 percent of the weight of the upper body is supported by the water volume that is stored in the disc core. And high blood pressure may be the result of an adaptive process to a gross body water deficiency. Drinking more water is a challenge for many people because they claim it's boring. Fresh juices provide an abundance of water, and can help you fulfill some of your much-needed water supply each day with delicious flavor.

JUICE RECIPES

Why not start your day with a glass of energizing juice? Instead of coffee midmorning, try a true pick-me-up with a fresh juice break. Any time of day, fresh juice offers one of the best sources of energy available. And it's so easy—especially with a good juicer (see page 9, "Choosing the Right Juicer") and some delicious recipes.

To make the nutrition information in this section as fun and accessible as possible, I've included "Nutrisips," tips on the nutritional benefits of one or more of the ingredients in a recipe. They will help you enjoy the recipes twice as much, knowing exactly how you are contributing to your own or someone else's well-being.

Keep in mind that some of the recipes are healthy tonics included in the last part of Vegetable-Fruit Juice Combinations. Not all of them are as tasty as others, but I encourage you to use them when they are recommended for your health. They can offer powerful components you'll get no other way.

Also, I have specified "organic" for all of the fruits and vegetables on the "dirty dozen" list. The nonprofit research organization Environmental Working Group reports periodically on health risks from pesticides in produce. The group says you can cut your pesticide exposure in half simply by avoiding the twelve conventionally grown fruits and vegetables found to be most contaminated. At this writing they are apples, apricots, bell peppers, celery, cherries, Chilean grapes, cucumbers, green beans, Mexican cantaloupes, peaches, spinach, and strawberries. However, organic is the healthiest choice for all fruits and vegetables.

VEGETABLE-FRUIT JUICE COMBINATIONS

I DRINK AT LEAST TWO big glasses (10 to 16 ounces) of vegetable-fruit combinations each day that I'm home and whenever I can find juice bars in other towns where I travel. Some of my favorite juice combinations are in this chapter—The Morning Energizer (page 16), Afternoon Refresher (page 18), Santa Fe Salsa Cocktail (page 19), and Parsley Pep (page 26; I omit the apple).

Most of the recipes in this chapter use some fruit for flavor, but the emphasis is on the vegetable juices. For your health, I recommend that you drink more vegetable juice than fruit juice. Also, some people, such as hypoglycemics, diabetics, and people with candidiasis, don't tolerate fruit juice well. I don't (due to hypoglycemia), and I typically use only lemon or lime for additional flavor. You can omit the fruit in any of the recipes in this chapter and you will still have delicious juice combinations. You also can add water to dilute any of the recipes that may be too strong-tasting or too high on the glycemic (sugars) index, such as carrot juice. Always dilute juices with water for children under the age of two, and never give juice to babies under six months old. (For more information, see Juicing for Babies and Children, page 136.)

The Morning Energizer

NUTRISIP: Beet juice is excellent to break the fast of the night before and cleanse the liver; beets have been used naturopathically to cleanse and support the liver for many years. Rich in vitamins and minerals that include beta carotene, zinc, vitamin C, and chromium, it is no wonder this drink is especially energizing.

½ Golden or Red Delicious organic apple, washed
5 medium carrots, scrubbed well, tops removed, ends trimmed
½ small beet with leaves and stems, scrubbed well
½ lemon, washed or peeled if not organic
½- to 1-inch piece ginger root, washed

Cut the apple into sections to fit your juicer's feed tube. Juice the apple with the carrots, beet, lemon, and ginger. Stir the juice and pour into a glass. Serve at room temperature or chilled, as desired.

Makes 12 to 14 ounces

Waldorf Twist

NUTRISIP: Celery juice has been used traditionally as a calming agent and to strengthen frayed nerves.

1 Red or Golden Delicious organic apple, washed
3 organic celery stalks with leaves, washed (see Note)
¼ lemon, washed or peeled if not organic

Cut the apple into sections that will fit your juicer's feed tube. Juice it with the celery and lemon. Stir the juice and pour into a glass. Serve at room temperature or chilled, as desired.

Makes about 8 ounces

Note: Do not store celery in the refrigerator for longer than three weeks. Studies show old celery has caused cancer in animals. Always discard wilted or brown celery.

The Ginger Hopper

NUTRISIP: Ginger has been shown in scientific studies to have anti-inflammatory properties.

½ Red or Golden Delicious organic apple, washed
5 medium carrots, scrubbed well, tops removed, ends trimmed
½- to 1-inch piece ginger root, washed

Cut the apple into sections that fit your juicer's feed tube. Juice it with the carrots and ginger. Stir the juice and pour into a glass. Serve at room temperature or chilled, as desired.

Makes about 8 ounces

Ginger Twist

NUTRISIP: Parsley is vitamin therapy all by itself. It is loaded with beta carotene, the precursor to vitamin A, and ounce for ounce, it has more than three times the vitamin C of an orange. In addition, it offers riboflavin (a B vitamin), calcium, iron, magnesium, and potassium. It is used traditionally as a diuretic.

1 Golden or Red Delicious organic apple, washed
1 small handful parsley, rinsed
4 carrots, scrubbed well, tops removed, ends trimmed
¼ lemon, washed or peeled if not organic
1-inch piece ginger root, washed

Cut the apple into sections that fit your juicer's feed tube. Bunch up the parsley and juice it with the apple, carrots, lemon, and ginger. Stir the juice and pour into a glass. Serve at room temperature or chilled, as desired.

Makes 8 to 10 ounces

Ginger Waldorf

NUTRISIP: Apples are rich in pectin, the soluble-type fiber that remains in the juice. It is speculated that the pectin works with other nutrients in the apple, like vitamin C, to carry cholesterol out of the blood.

2 large Golden or Red Delicious organic apples, washed
3 organic celery stalks with leaves, washed (see Note)
1/2-inch piece ginger root, washed

Cut the apples into sections that fit your juicer's feed tube. Juice the apples with the celery and ginger. Stir the juice and pour into a glass. Serve at room temperature or chilled, as desired.

Makes about 10 ounces

Note: Do not store celery in the refrigerator for longer than three weeks. Studies show that old celery has caused cancer in animals. Always discard wilted or brown celery.

Afternoon Refresher

NUTRISIP: Cucumbers are among nature's most effective diuretics. They are also great thirst quenchers. Caravan travelers often carried cucumbers on desert travels in the Middle East to refresh the body and satisfy thirst.

1 medium to large organic cucumber, washed or peeled if not organic
1/2 lemon, washed or peeled if not organic

Cut the cucumber lengthwise in half and juice with the lemon. For an especially cooling version, let the juice splash over ice cubes in a pitcher. Stir the juice and pour into a glass. Serve chilled or at room temperature.

Makes 8 to 10 ounces

Orient Express

NUTRISIP: In traditional Oriental medicine, daikon-carrot drinks are used to help eliminate fats and dissolve hardened accumulations in the intestines.

2-inch length jicama, scrubbed or peeled if not organic
5 medium carrots, scrubbed well, tops removed, ends trimmed
2-inch length daikon radish, trimmed, if necessary, and scrubbed
1/2- to 1-inch piece ginger root, washed

Cut jicama into strips that will fit your juicer's feed tube. Juice the jicama with the carrots, daikon, and ginger root. Stir the juice and pour into a glass. Serve at room temperature or chilled, as desired.

Makes 12 to 14 ounces

Santa Fe Salsa Cocktail

NUTRISIP: Lycopene is an antioxidant that gives tomatoes their bright red color; it appears to be twice as powerful an antioxidant as beta carotene.

1 medium vine-ripened organic tomato, washed
½ medium cucumber, washed and peeled if not organic
1 small handful cilantro, rinsed
¼ lime, washed or peeled if not organic
Dash of hot sauce (optional)

Cut the tomato into sections that will fit your juicer's feed tube. Cut the cucumber lengthwise in half. Bunch up the cilantro and juice it with the tomato, cucumber, and lime. Pour the juice into a glass, add the hot sauce, and mix well. Serve at room temperature or chilled, as desired.

Makes 8 to 10 ounces

Spicy Tomato on Ice

NUTRISIP: One study has shown that tomatoes can help protect the body against acute appendicitis.

2 medium vine-ripened tomatoes, washed
2 dark green lettuce leaves, washed
2 radishes, washed
5 parsley sprigs, rinsed
½ lime or lemon, washed or peeled if not organic
Dash of hot sauce

Cut the tomato into sections that will fit your juicer's feed tube. Bunch up the lettuce leaves and parsley and juice them with the tomatoes, radishes, and lime or lemon. Add the hot sauce and stir the juice. Pour into an ice-filled glass.

Makes about 10 ounces

Morning Express

NUTRISIP: Oranges offer selenium, a mineral that has been shown in studies to have powerful antioxidant effects.

1 orange, peeled
4 to 5 carrots, scrubbed well, tops removed, ends trimmed

Divide the orange into segments that will fit your juicer's feed tube. Juice the orange with the carrots. Stir the juice and pour into a glass. Serve at room temperature or chilled, as desired.

Makes about 8 ounces

Triple C

NUTRISIP: Cabbage and its cruciferous family, which includes broccoli, Brussels sprouts, and cauliflower, are esteemed for their cancer-preventive properties. Research shows that they contain various phytochemicals, including chlorophyll, indole, and isothiocyanates, which help detoxify the system and strengthen the immune cells.

¼ small head of green cabbage, washed
4 carrots, scrubbed well, tops removed, ends trimmed
4 organic celery stalks with leaves, washed (see Note, page 18)

Cut the cabbage into sections that will fit your juicer's feed tube. Juice the cabbage with the carrots and celery. Stir the juice and pour into a glass. Serve at room temperature or chilled, as desired.

Makes 8 to 10 ounces

Popeye's Power

NUTRISIP: Nutritional surveys show that consuming as little a one-half cup of spinach per day may cut the risk of cancer, especially of the lungs, almost in half. One scientist found spinach juice to be the most potent of the five foods tested (carrot, cauliflower, lettuce, spinach, and strawberry) in blocking highly carcinogenic nitrosamines.

> $^1/_2$ medium organic apple, washed
> 1 handful organic spinach, rinsed
> 4 medium carrots, scrubbed well, tops removed, ends trimmed
> 1 organic celery stalk with leaves, washed (see Note, page 18)
> $^1/_2$ beet with leaves, scrubbed well
> 1 small handful parsley, rinsed

Cut the apple into sections that will fit your juicer's feed tube. Bunch up the spinach and juice it with the apple, carrots, celery, beet, and parsley. Stir the juice and pour into a glass. Serve at room temperature or chilled, as desired.

Makes about 10 ounces

Wheatgrass Light

NUTRISIP: You may need to develop a taste for wheatgrass, but whether you do or not, include it in your juice diet for all its healthful benefits. Wheatgrass is rich in chlorophyll, a phytonutrient that gives plants their green color; chlorophyll is a blood purifier. You could also consider it concentrated "sun power"—the same energy source that enables clumps of grass to push their way through sidewalks.

> 1 Golden or Red Delicious organic apple, washed
> 1 small handful wheatgrass, rinsed
> 2 to 3 mint sprigs, rinsed (optional)
> $^1/_4$ lemon, washed or peeled if not organic

Cut the apple into sections that will fit your juicer's feed tube. Bunch up the wheatgrass and mint, and juice them with the apple and lemon. Stir the juice and pour into a glass. Serve at room temperature or chilled, as desired.

Makes about 8 ounces

Tomato Florentine

NUTRISIP: Tomato is a source of tyramine, which is a precursor to tyrosine, an amino acid. Thyroid hormones are made from iodine and tyrosine; therefore, it follows that tomatoes help promote thyroid balance.

2 vine-ripened tomatoes, washed
1 handful organic spinach, washed
Several basil sprigs (optional)
$\frac{1}{2}$ lemon, washed or peeled if not organic

Cut the tomatoes in half. Bunch up the spinach and basil, as desired, and juice them with the tomatoes and lemon. Pour the juice into a glass and stir. Serve at room temperature or chilled, as desired.

Makes 8 to 10 ounces

Pure Green Sprout Drink

NUTRISIP: Sprouts give us the most concentrated natural sources of vitamins, minerals, enzymes, and amino acids available, along with bioelectrical energy. They are considered one of nature's most perfect foods.

1 organic cucumber, scrubbed well or peeled if not organic
1 large handful sunflower sprouts
1 small handful buckwheat sprouts
1 small handful clover sprouts

Cut the cucumber lengthwise in half and juice it with the sprouts. Stir to combine and serve at room temperature.

Makes about 8 ounces

Magnesium Special

NUTRISIP: Carrots, beets, celery, and broccoli are all good sources of magnesium, which is important for protein synthesis. Magnesium can make a significant difference in strength training.

5 medium carrots, scrubbed well, tops removed, ends trimmed
2 organic celery stalks, with leaves, washed (see Note, page 18)

½ small beet with leaves and stems, scrubbed well
2 broccoli florets, washed
½ lemon, washed or peeled if not organic

Juice the carrots, celery, beet, broccoli, and lemon. Stir the juice and pour into a glass. Serve at room temperature or chilled, as desired.

Makes about 12 ounces

Mint Medley

NUTRISIP: Fennel has been used traditionally to promote digestion and relieve gas.

2 organic apples (any variety), washed
2 fennel stalks with leaves, washed
1 small handful mint, washed
½-inch piece of ginger, washed

Cut the apples into sections that will fit your juicer's feed tube. Juice the apples with the fennel, mint, and ginger. Pour the juice into a glass and stir. Serve at room temperature or chilled, as desired.

Makes 10 to 12 ounces

Orange Velvet

NUTRISIP: Orange juice is rich in vitamin C and also is high in folic acid as well as selenium. Folic acid is required for DNA synthesis and cell replication and is recommended for pregnant women to help prevent neural tube defects.

½ small jicama, scrubbed well or peeled if not organic
1 orange, peeled
¼ lime, washed or peeled if not organic

Cut the jicama and the orange into sections that will fit your juicer's feed tube. Juice the jicama and orange with the lime. Stir the juice and pour into a glass. Serve at room temperature or chilled, as desired.

Makes 8 ounces

Sweet Calcium Cocktail

NUTRISIP: If you have trouble getting your children to eat calcium-rich foods or if someone in your family is dairy sensitive, try mixing kale, one of the best sources of calcium, with pineapple juice.

3-inch chunk of fresh pineapple, scrubbed well or peeled if not organic
1 to 2 kale leaves, washed

Cut the pineapple into strips that will fit your juicer's feed tube. Bunch up the kale, tuck it into the feed tube, and juice it with the pineapple. Stir the juice and pour into a glass. Serve at room temperature or chilled, as desired.

Makes about 8 ounces

Beautiful Skin, Hair, and Nails Cocktail

NUTRISIP: Cucumber and bell pepper are good sources of silicon, which is known as the beauty nutrient. Silicon is recommended to strengthen bones, skin, hair, and fingernails. In one study, women who showed visible signs of aging of their facial skin, fragile hair, and brittle nails, and who took supplemental silicon (colloidal silicic acid), showed significant improved thickness and strength of skin, diminished wrinkles, and healthier hair and nails. In addition, parsnip juice is a traditional remedy for beautifying skin, hair, and nails; drink one cup every day to improve and maintain beautiful skin, hair, and nails.

1 medium organic cucumber, washed or peeled if not organic
1 medium parsnip, scrubbed well
3 medium carrots, scrubbed well, tops removed, ends trimmed
½ lemon, peeled if not organic
¼ small organic green bell pepper, washed

Cut the cucumber and parsnip lengthwise in half. Juice the cucumber and parsnip with the carrots, lemon, and bell pepper. Stir the juice and pour into a glass. Serve at room temperature or chilled, as desired.

Makes about 16 ounces

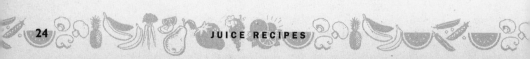

Refreshing Complexion Cocktail

NUTRISIP: Cucumber juice has been used as a traditional remedy to reduce acne problems and diminish facial wrinkles. Since the days of Cleopatra, cucumber has been known to work wonders for the skin.

½ Golden or Red Delicious organic apple, washed
2-inch chunk of pineapple, washed or peeled if not organic
1 medium organic cucumber, washed or peeled if not organic

Cut the apple into sections and the pineapple into strips that will fit your juicer's feed tube. Cut the cucumber lengthwise. Juice the apple, pineapple, and cucumber. Stir the juice and pour into a glass. Serve at room temperature or chilled, as desired.

Makes about 12 ounces

Beautiful Bone Solution

NUTRISIP: Kale and parsley top the list of calcium-rich foods, ounce for ounce beating milk by about a two-to-one ratio. They also are excellent sources of vitamin K, which helps anchor calcium in bones; magnesium, which works with calcium to strengthen bones; and the trace mineral boron, which reduces calcium excretion.

1 Golden or Red Delicious organic apple, washed
1 to 2 medium-large kale leaves, washed
1 handful parsley, washed
1 organic celery stalk, washed (see Note, page 18)
¼ lemon, washed or peeled if not organic
½- to 1-inch piece ginger root, washed

Section the apple to fit into your juicer's feed tube. Bunch up the kale and parsley and juice them with the apple, celery, lemon, and ginger. Stir the juice and pour into a glass. Serve at room temperature or chilled, as desired.

Makes 8 to 10 ounces

Parsley Pep

NUTRISIP: Parsley is a traditional remedy to increase energy.

1 bunch parsley, washed
2 organic celery stalks, washed (see Note, page 18)
1 to 2 carrots, scrubbed well, tops removed, ends trimmed
¼ to ½ lemon, washed or peeled if not organic

Bunch up the parsley and tuck it in the feed tube; juice with the celery, carrots, and lemon. Stir the juice and pour into a glass. Serve at room temperature or chilled, as desired.

Makes 6 to 8 ounces

Digestive Tonic

NUTRISIP: This juice combination has been used traditionally for weak digestive systems. Drink a glass of this tonic in the morning and evening.

½ pear, washed
5 carrots, scrubbed well, tops removed, ends trimmed
¼ medium jicama, scrubbed well or peeled if not organic

Cut the pear into sections that will fit your juicer's feed tube. Juice the pear with the carrots and jicama. Stir the juice and pour into a glass. For a weak digestive system or if you have a lung condition, serve this juice at room temperature (chilled is too hard on weak lungs and a compromised intestinal tract); otherwise, serve chilled, if desired.

Makes 8 to 10 ounces

The Colon Cleanser

NUTRISIP: Apple and spinach juice have been used as a traditional remedy for cleansing the colon. Drink two 8-ounce glasses (one in the morning and one in the evening) of this cocktail per day on an empty stomach for five to seven days. Also this is an effective colon mover.

2 Granny Smith, McIntosh, or Golden Delicious organic apples,
   washed

1 bunch organic spinach, washed well
1 handful parsley, washed
¼ lemon, washed or peeled if not organic

Cut the apples into sections. Bunch up the spinach and parsley, tuck them in the feed tube, and juice them with the apples and lemon. Stir the juice and pour into a glass. Serve at room temperature or chilled, as desired.

Makes about 8 to 10 ounces

The Gallbladder Cleansing Cocktail

NUTRISIP: Traditionally, carrot, beet, and cucumber juices have been used to cleanse the liver, gallbladder, and kidneys. For the gallbladder, drink this combination three to four times a day along with several glasses of lemon juice in hot water; this has helped many people dissolve gallstones in a few days to several weeks.

4 carrots, scrubbed well, tops removed, ends trimmed
½ organic cucumber, washed or peeled if not organic
½ medium beet with greens, scrubbed well
¼ lemon, washed or peeled if not organic

Juice the carrots, cucumber, beet, and lemon. Stir the juice and pour into a glass. Serve at room temperature or chilled, as desired.

Makes about 10 ounces

The Memory Mender

NUTRISIP: Iceberg lettuce, cauliflower, and tomato are good sources of choline. Choline increases the accumulation within the brain of acetylcholine, an important chemical utilized in a variety of brain processes. Some evidence exists that increasing brain acetylcholine by supplementing choline results in improved memory.

2 medium vine-ripened tomatoes, washed
¼ small head of iceberg lettuce, washed
4 cauliflower florets, washed
½ lemon, washed or peeled if not organic

Cut the tomatoes and lettuce into sections that will fit your juicer's feed tube. Juice the tomato and lettuce with the cauliflower and lemon. Stir the juice and pour into a glass. Serve at room temperature or chilled, as desired.

Makes 8 to 10 ounces

Hangover Helper

NUTRISIP: The liver is adversely impacted by overconsumption of alcohol. Tomato juice combined with string bean juice and a dash of hot sauce will help to revitalize the liver and improve vitality. Alcohol also is very dehydrating; this juice combination will help to rehydrate the body quickly.

2 medium to large vine-ripened tomatoes, washed
½ organic cucumber, washed or peeled if not organic
6 organic string beans, washed
¼ lime or lemon, washed or peeled if not organic
Dash of hot sauce

Cut the tomatoes into sections that will fit your juicer's feed tube and cut the cucumber lengthwise in half. Juice the tomatoes, cucumber, string beans, and lime or lemon. Pour the juice into a glass, add the hot sauce, and stir until well mixed. Serve at room temperature or chilled, as desired.

Makes 10 to 12 ounces

Weight-Loss Express

NUTRISIP: Ginger is thermogenic, meaning it helps produce body heat and thus burns calories. Cucumbers and parsley are natural diuretics that can help rid the body of excess water.

½ organic cucumber, washed or peeled if not organic
½ large pippin or Granny Smith organic apple, washed
4 to 5 carrots, scrubbed well, tops removed, ends trimmed
1 small handful parsley, rinsed
½ lemon, washed or peeled if not organic
1-inch piece ginger root, washed

Halve the cucumber lengthwise; cut the apple into sections to fit your juicer's feed tube. Juice all the ingredients. Stir the juice and pour into a glass. Serve at room temperature or chilled, as desired.

Makes 10 to 12 ounces

Weight-Loss Buddy

NUTRISIP: Jerusalem artichoke juice combined with carrot and beet is a traditional remedy for satisfying cravings for sweets and junk food. The key is to sip this drink slowly when you have a craving for high-fat or high-sugar foods.

1 small Jerusalem artichoke, scrubbed well
4 medium carrots, scrubbed well, tops removed, ends trimmed
½ small beet, scrubbed well, top removed

Cut the artichoke into pieces that will fit your juicer's feed tube. Juice the artichoke with the carrots and beet. Stir the juice and pour into a glass. Serve at room temperature or chilled, as desired.

Makes 8 to 10 ounces

Sweet Dreams Nightcap

NUTRISIP: A deficiency of calcium and magnesium can cause you to wake up in the middle of the night and not be able to drift off to sleep again; parsley, carrot, and celery are good sources of these minerals. This nightcap also contains some of the B vitamins that help promote a restful state. Romaine lettuce has been observed to have some sedative effects and celery to have calming effects.

2 romaine lettuce leaves, washed
1 small handful parsley, washed
4 carrots, scrubbed well, tops removed, ends trimmed
3 organic celery stalks with leaves, washed (see Note, page 18)

Bunch up the lettuce and parsley and tuck them in the feed tube; juice with the carrots and celery. Stir the juice and pour into a glass. Serve at room temperature or chilled, as desired.

Makes about 8 ounces

The Feel-Good Cocktail

NUTRISIP: Fennel juice has been used as a traditional tonic to help release endorphins, the feel-good peptides, from the brain into the bloodstream. Endorphins create a mood of euphoria and help dampen anxiety and fear.

½ pear, washed
4 medium carrots, scrubbed well, tops removed, ends trimmed
3 fennel stalks with leaves and flowers, washed
1 organic celery stalk with leaves, washed (see Note, page 18)

Cut the pear into sections that will fit your juicer's feed tube. Juice the pear with the carrots, fennel, and celery. Stir the juice and pour into a glass. Serve at room temperature or chilled, as desired.

Makes 10 to 12 ounces

Radish Solution

NUTRISIP: Radish juice is a traditional remedy to open sinus cavities and strengthen mucous membranes.

2 medium vine-ripened tomatoes, washed
4 radishes with tops, washed
¼ lime or lemon, washed or peeled if not organic

Cut the tomato into sections that will fit your juicer's feed tube. Juice the tomatoes with the radishes and lime or lemon. Stir the juice and pour into a glass. Serve at room temperature or chilled, as desired.

Makes about 8 ounces

The Immune Builder

NUTRISIP: Studies have shown garlic's smelly compound, allicin, to have a natural antibiotic effect. Garlic is antibacterial, antifungal, antiparasitic, and antiviral. Garlic must be raw to have an antibiotic effect; once it is cooked, it is no longer a microbe destroyer. Apple juice also has shown antiviral effects when studied in test tubes.

1 medium Golden or Red Delicious organic apple, washed
1 turnip, scrubbed well
1 handful watercress, washed
5 medium carrots, scrubbed well, tops removed, ends trimmed
1 large garlic clove with peel, washed

Cut the apple and turnip into sections that will fit your juicer's feed tube. Bunch up the watercress, tuck it in the feed tube, and juice the apple and turnip with the watercress, carrots, and garlic. Stir the juice and pour into a glass. Serve at room temperature or chilled, as desired.

Makes about 10 ounces

Jack and the Bean

NUTRISIP: Brussels sprout and string bean juice have been used as traditional remedies to help strengthen and regenerate the pancreas. Drink four ounces before each meal. This remedy works best when sugars (including fruit) and most starches are avoided. This combination is quite strong-tasting; dilute with water as desired.

1 large tomato, washed
2 romaine lettuce leaves, washed
8 organic string beans, washed
5 Brussels sprouts, washed
½ lemon, washed or peeled if not organic

Cut the tomatoes into sections that will fit your juicer's feed tube. Bunch up the lettuce leaves and put them in the juicer first, followed by some of the tomato sections. Juice the remaining tomato with the string beans, Brussels sprouts, and lemon. Stir the juice and pour into a glass. Serve at room temperature or chilled, as desired.

Makes about 10 ounces

Radish Care

NUTRISIP: Radish juice has been used as a traditional remedy to promote a healthy thyroid.

5 carrots, scrubbed well, tops removed, ends trimmed
5 to 6 radishes with tops, washed well
1/2 lemon, washed or peeled if not organic

Juice the carrots, radishes, and lemon. Stir the juice and pour into a glass. Serve at room temperature or chilled, as desired.

Makes about 8 ounces

Turnip Time

NUTRISIP: Turnips have been used as a traditional remedy to strengthen the lungs. To promote healthy lungs, drink two 8-ounce glasses with meals daily.

1 small turnip, scrubbed well
2-inch-length jicama, scrubbed well or peeled if not organic (optional)
1 handful watercress, rinsed
4 carrots, scrubbed well, tops removed, ends trimmed
1 garlic clove with peel, washed
1/2 lemon, washed or peeled if not organic

Cut the turnip and jicama into pieces that will fit your juicer's feed tube. Bunch up the watercress and juice it with the turnip, jicama (if using), watercress, carrots, garlic, and lemon. Stir the juice and pour into a glass. Serve at room temperature or chilled, as desired. If you have weakened lungs, drink this at room temperature only; chilled drinks are too hard on weak lungs. You may want to dilute this drink with at least $\frac{1}{2}$ cup water since the turnip juice is quite strong and distinct-tasting.

Makes 16 ounces

Spring Tonic

NUTRISIP: Asparagus juice is a traditional remedy to promote healthy kidneys and prostate glands. Asparagus juice also is a natural diuretic. Juice the stems and use the tips, lightly steamed or grilled, with a meal.

1 medium vine-ripened tomato, washed
1 organic cucumber, washed or peeled if not organic
8 asparagus stems, washed
$\frac{1}{2}$ small lemon, washed or peeled if not organic

Cut the tomato into sections that will fit your juicer's feed tube. Cut the cucumber lengthwise in half. Juice the tomato, cucumber, asparagus, and lemon. Stir the juice and pour into a glass. Serve at room temperature or chilled, as desired.

Makes 10 to 12 ounces

Liver Life Cocktail

NUTRISIP: Dandelion juice has been used traditionally to cleanse the liver. Dandelion juice is very strong and somewhat bitter-tasting. You may want to dilute this drink with some water. (Don't pick any dandelion leaves unless you absolutely know that they have not been sprayed; many yard sprays contain arsenic.)

On a personal note, my grandmother often made a spring tonic by boiling dandelion leaves and drinking the tea. I can still picture her picking dandelion leaves in our backyard. Having practiced natural medicines on herself all her life, she was rarely ill and died at the age of 94. I believe her dandelion tea was one of her health secrets.

½ small green organic apple, such as Granny Smith or pippin, washed
1 handful organic dandelion greens, washed
5 carrots, scrubbed well, tops removed, ends trimmed
½ small lemon, washed or peeled if not organic

Cut the apple into wedges that will fit your juicer's feed tube. Juice the apple with the dandelion greens, carrots, and lemon. Stir the juice and pour into a glass. Serve at room temperature or chilled, as desired.

Makes 8 to 10 ounces

FRUIT JUICE RECIPES

FRUITS (AND VEGETABLES) RANK AMONG our best sources of beta carotene (provitamin A) and vitamin C—two important disease-fighting antioxidants. Just how important is it to get plenty of these nutrients? *Medical World News* (1993) reported on a 12-year Swiss study of 3,000 men; it found that low serum levels of beta carotene and vitamin A were highly correlated with an increased risk of lung cancer and death from all forms of cancer. Hundreds of other studies show vitamin C along with beta carotene to be protective against cancer.

The National Cancer Institute Guidelines encourage eating two to four servings of fruit per day and three to five servings of vegetables. It was found, however, in the National Health and Nutrition examination (INHANES II) that a one-day look at the diet of 12,000 Americans showed that 41 percent ate no fruit on that survey day and only 25 percent reported eating a fruit or vegetable rich in provitamin A (beta carotene) or vitamin C.

Juicing fruits offers advantages to busy people who find it difficult to get all the recommended servings of fruits (and vegetables) each day. Juicing is fast, easy, and convenient and is one way Americans can make sure they are getting the two to four fruit servings each day.

Fruit juices are the energizers and cleansers of the body; citrus juices are especially cleansing. Some fruits, such as pineapple, kiwi, and papaya, assist digestion. Others have been shown in scientific studies to help heal the body, such as cranberry juice for bladder infections.

People with diabetes or hypoglycemia should be aware that fruit juice is high in fruit sugar and should be avoided or consumed in very small quantities diluted with water. Also, people with candidiasis should avoid fruit and fruit juice completely. If you are challenged with any of these conditions, I recommend that you avoid this section and choose your juices from the vegetable-fruit juice section. Even from that section I suggest that you omit all fruits except for lemon and lime.

Apple Spice

NUTRISIP: Does an apple a day keep the doctor away? There are researchers who will tell you that viruses don't live very long when introduced to apple juice or grape juice. When researchers poured apple juice into test tubes, it rendered polioviruses inactive. If you don't have time to eat your apple a day, don't forget to drink it.

1 large organic apple (any variety), washed
1 bunch green or red (organic if Chilean) grapes, washed
$1/2$- to 1-inch piece ginger root, washed

Cut the apple into sections that will fit your juicer's feed tube. Juice the apple with the grapes and ginger. Stir the juice and pour into a glass. Serve at room temperature or chilled, as desired.

Makes about 8 ounces

Sweet and Regular

NUTRISIP: The pectins (water-soluble fiber) in pears and apples cleanse the body of toxins and wastes and help improve peristaltic action in the intestines, which helps to keep us regular.

2 pears (any variety), washed
1 organic apple (any variety), washed

Cut the pears and apple into sections that will fit your juicer's feed tube. Juice the pears and apple. Pour the juice into a glass and stir. Serve at room temperature or chilled, as desired.

Makes 8 ounces

Pink Lemonade

NUTRISIP: Lemons are a good source of bioflavonoids—phytonutrients that enhance the effectiveness of vitamin C. They help reduce capillary fragility, thus reducing easy bruising and swelling and bruising after sports injuries.

2 to 3 medium to large Golden or Red Delicious organic apples, washed
1/4 lemon, washed or peeled if not organic
1/2-inch cube beet, scrubbed well (added for color)

Cut the apples into sections that will fit your juicer's feed tube. Juice the apples with the lemon and beet. Stir the juice and pour into an ice-filled glass, or let the juice splash over ice in the juice pitcher. Serve chilled.

Makes about 8 ounces

Just Peachy

NUTRISIP: The combination of peach and pear juices is a traditional remedy that helps promote healthy lungs.

1 organic peach, washed, stone removed, peeled if not organic
1 pear with core, washed, peeled if not organic
1/2- to 1-inch piece ginger root, washed

Cut the peach and pear into sections that will fit your juicer's feed tube. Juice the peach, pear, and ginger. Stir the juice, pour into a glass, and serve at room temperature for lung conditions (cold foods are too hard on weak lungs), or chilled, as desired, if a lung condition is not of concern.

Makes about 8 ounces

Strawberry-Cantaloupe Cocktail

NUTRISIP: Cantaloupe is a good source of carotenoids. Hundreds of studies from around the world point to carotenes having cancer-preventive properties. Cantaloupe, with seeds, also is a natural diuretic.

*1/2 ripe (organic if Mexican) cantaloupe with seeds,
    washed or peeled if not organic*
1 cup organic strawberries with caps, washed

Cut the cantaloupe into strips that will fit your juicer's feed tube. Juice the cantaloupe and strawberries. Stir the juice and pour into a glass. Serve at room temperature or chilled, as desired.

Makes about 16 ounces

Snappy Ginger

NUTRISIP: Ginger helps prevent motion sickness and nausea. It has been effective for women suffering from morning sickness.

1 medium orange, peeled
3-inch chunk of pineapple, scrubbed well or peeled if not organic
1/4 lemon, washed or peeled if not organic
1- to 2-inch piece ginger root, washed

Divide the orange into sections and the pineapple into strips that will fit your juicer's feed tube. Juice the orange, pineapple, lemon, and ginger. Stir the juice and pour into 2 glasses. Serve at room temperature or chilled, as desired.

Makes about 16 ounces

Cranberry-Apple Cocktail

NUTRISIP: A number of studies have shown that cranberry juice is effective in promoting healthy urinary tracts.

2 to 3 medium Golden or Red Delicious organic apples, washed
1/2 cup fresh or frozen (thawed) cranberries, rinsed
1/2 lemon, washed or peeled if not organic

Cut the apples into sections that will fit your juicer's feed tube. To prevent the cranberries from flying out of the machine while juicing, turn it off before putting the cranberries in the machine. Place the cranberries in the juicer first and then put a piece of apple on top of them and the plunger on top of the apple. Turn on the machine and push the plunger to begin the juicing process. Juice the remaining apple with the lemon. Stir the juice and pour into a glass. Serve at room temperature or chilled, as desired.

Makes 8 to 10 ounces

Antiaging Solution

NUTRISIP: Deep purple grapes and berries are a source of anthocyanidins and proanthocyanidins, phytonutrients that help to stabilize collagen structures, thus preventing a loss of the skin's elasticity.

> *1 small bunch (about 1 cup) purple (organic if Chilean) grapes with*
> *   small stems and seeds, washed (remove large stems, which can dull*
> *   the juicer blade)*
> *½ cup blueberries, blackberries, or raspberries, washed*
> *¼ lemon, washed or peeled if not organic*
> *½-inch piece fresh ginger root, washed*

Juice the grapes, berries, lemon, and ginger. Stir the juice and pour into a glass. Serve at room temperature or chilled, as desired.

Makes about 8 ounces

Morning Sunrise

NUTRISIP: This drink also could be called "the fat burner." The white pithy part of the grapefruit and orange, located just beneath the peel, is a rich source of bioflavonoids—particularly hesperidin and rutin—which, according to folk remedy, help to burn excess fat.

> *1 pink, red, or white grapefruit, peeled*
> *1 orange, peeled*

Cut the grapefruit and orange into sections that will fit your juicer's feed tube. Juice the grapefruit and orange and stir the juice. Pour into a glass and serve at room temperature or chilled, as desired.

Makes 8 to 10 ounces

Grape Expectations

NUTRISIP: Two recent studies indicate that drinking three glasses of grape juice a day reduces platelet aggregation (clotting) by 40 percent, thus promoting a healthy heart.

3 plums, washed, stones removed (optional)
$\frac{1}{2}$ pound purple (organic if Chilean) grapes with seeds and small stems
    (remove large stems as they can dull the juicer blade)
8 organic strawberries with caps or $\frac{1}{2}$ sweet organic apple, washed
$\frac{1}{4}$ lemon, washed or peeled if not organic

Cut the plums (if using) in half and juice them with the grapes, strawberries or apple, and lemon. Stir the juice and pour into a glass. Serve at room temperature or chilled, as desired.

Makes about 10 ounces

Watermelon Refresher

NUTRISIP: Watermelon is considered a natural diuretic. Juice the seeds and rind, too. The seeds are believed to have a high concentration of diuretic properties, and the rind contains chlorophyll, a blood purifier.

1-inch-thick slice of watermelon with seeds and rind,
    rind scrubbed well

Cut the watermelon into pieces that will fit your juicer's feed tube. Juice the watermelon and pour into a glass. Serve at room temperature or chilled, as desired.

Makes 12 to 16 ounces

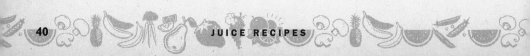

Tangerine Squeeze

NUTRISIP: Chinese traditional medicine uses tangerine juice to prevent mucous congestion in the throat, sinuses, and lungs. Citrus juices also are good to help cleanse the liver.

1/4 ripe pineapple with core, scrubbed well or peeled if not organic
2 to 3 tangerines, peeled
1/4 lime, washed or peeled if not organic

Cut the pineapple into pieces and the tangerine into sections that will fit your juicer's feed tube. Juice the pineapple, tangerines, and lime. Stir the juice and pour into a glass. Serve at room temperature or chilled, as desired.

Makes 8 to 10 ounces

Tropical Treat

NUTRISIP: Kiwifruit has natural diuretic properties, making it a good weight-loss helper. Also, it is said to help facilitate the removal of excess sodium.

2 firm kiwifruits, washed or peeled if not organic
1 small green organic apple (any variety), washed
1-inch chunk of ripe pineapple, scrubbed well or peeled if not organic
1/2-inch piece fresh ginger root, washed

Cut the kiwis, apple, and pineapple into pieces that will fit your juicer's feed tube. Juice the kiwis, apple, pineapple, and ginger. Stir to combine the juice and pour into a glass. Serve at room temperature or chilled, as desired.

Makes 8 to 10 ounces

Tropical Spice

NUTRISIP: Ginger root is warming and stimulating; it promotes gastric secretions and aids in the absorption of nutrients.

3-inch chunk of pineapple, scrubbed well or peeled if not organic
1 kiwifruit, washed
1 small handful mint, washed
¹/₂-inch piece of ginger root, washed

Cut the pineapple into strips that will fit your juicer's feed tube. Cut the kiwi in half. Juice the pineapple, kiwi, mint, and ginger. Pour the juice into a glass and stir. Serve at room temperature or chilled, as desired.

Makes 10 to 12 ounces

Cherry Jubilee

NUTRISIP: Cherry juice is a traditional remedy to help cleanse the body. This can be quite beneficial for people who suffer from skin problems that are due to toxins and waste matter that has accumulated in the system.

3-inch chunk of ripe pineapple, scrubbed well or peeled if not organic
¹/₂ Golden or Red Delicious organic apple, washed
6 to 8 organic Bing cherries, washed and pitted

Cut the pineapple and apple into pieces that will fit your juicer's feed tube. Juice the pineapple and apple with the cherries; stir the juice and pour into a glass. Serve at room temperature or chilled, as desired.

Makes about 8 ounces

Pink Passion Potion

NUTRISIP: Cranberries are a traditional remedy for cleansing the kidneys.

1 Red Delicious organic apple, washed
1 bunch purple (organic if Chilean) grapes with seeds and small stems, washed (remove large stems, which can dull the juicer's blade)
¹/₂ cup fresh or frozen (thawed) cranberries, rinsed

½-inch piece beet (optional, for color)
¼ lemon, washed or peeled if not organic

Cut the apple into pieces that will fit your juicer's feed tube. Pick single grapes and small grape clusters off the larger stems. Start with your machine turned off. Add the cranberries, place an apple piece on top, followed by the plunger. Turn on the machine. Juice the remaining apple, grapes, and lemon; stir the juice and pour into a glass. Serve at room temperature or chilled, as desired.

Makes 8 to 10 ounces

After-Dinner Mint

NUTRISIP: Mint is good for digestion because it has demonstrated an antispasmodic effect on smooth muscle like that of the digestive system. Kiwifruit also is a digestive helper; like papaya and pineapple, it contains enzymes that aid digestion. This drink is beneficial after dinner, especially a heavy meal, to help relieve the feeling of fullness.

2 firm kiwifruits with skin, washed or peeled if not organic
1 large Golden Delicious organic apple, washed
1 small handful mint, rinsed

Cut the kiwis and apple into pieces that will fit your juicer's feed tube. Bunch up the mint, tuck it in the feed tube, and juice it with the apple and kiwis; stir the juice and pour into a glass. Serve at room temperature or chilled, as desired.

Makes about 8 ounces

Raspberry Sunrise

NUTRISIP: Raspberries are a rich source of anthocyanidins and proanthocyanidins—phytonutrients that stabilize the integrity and structure of collagen, which is the major protein structure not only in skin, but also in bone.

1 orange, peeled
1 Golden or Red Delicious organic apple, washed
1 pint raspberries, rinsed

Cut the orange and apple into pieces that will fit your juicer's feed tube. Juice the orange and apple with the raspberries; stir the juice and pour into a glass. Serve at room temperature or chilled, as desired.

Makes about 12 ounces

Apricot Nectar

NUTRISIP: Apricots are a rich source of beta carotene (provitamin A), which helps protect the skin from ultraviolet sun rays.

4 organic apricots, stones removed, washed
1 large Golden or Red Delicious organic apple, washed

Cut the apple into sections that will fit your juicer's feed tube. Juice the apple and apricots and stir the juice. Pour into a glass and serve at room temperature or chilled, as desired.

Makes about 8 ounces

Strawberry Lemonade

NUTRISIP: A 1997 study done with eight elderly women who were given strawberry beverages found a 20 percent increase in their serum antioxidant capacity. This was equivalent to taking 1,250 mg of vitamin C.

3 medium Golden or Red Delicious organic apples, washed
1 cup organic strawberries, with caps, washed
½ lemon, washed or peeled if not organic

Cut the apples into sections that will fit your juicer's feed tube. Juice the apples with the strawberries and lemon. Stir the juice and pour into 2 ice-filled glasses, or let the juice splash over ice in the juice pitcher. Serve chilled.

Makes about 16 ounces

Sweet Summertime in the Tropics

NUTRISIP: Pineapple is rich in the enzyme bromelain, which is beneficial to digestion.

> *3-inch chunk of pineapple, scrubbed well or peeled if not organic*
> *1 kiwifruit, washed or peeled if not organic*
> *¼ lime, washed or peeled if not organic*
> *½ cup low-fat coconut milk (optional)*

Cut the pineapple into pieces that will fit your juicer's feed tube. Cut the kiwi in half. Juice the pineapple, kiwi, and lime. Add the coconut milk, if desired, and stir the juice well. Pour it into 2 ice-filled glasses for a summertime treat.

Makes about 16 ounces

Minty Melon Cooler

NUTRISIP: Melons have been shown in scientific studies to thin the blood. Researchers identified the anticoagulant in melon as adenosine, which is also present in onions and garlic. All three foods are excellent to help promote a healthy heart.

> *½ medium honeydew melon, washed or peeled if not organic*
> *1 bunch fresh mint (about 1 cup, packed), rinsed*

Cut the melon into strips that will fit your juicer's feed tube. Bunch up the mint and juice it with the melon. Place some ice cubes in the juice pitcher and let the juice splash over the ice for a cool, refreshing drink. Stir the juice and pour into 2 glasses. Serve chilled.

Makes about 16 ounces

Pineapple Express

NUTRISIP: Pineapple contains bromelain, an enzyme that has well-documented effectiveness in fighting inflammation. This also is an excellent combination for scratchy throats.

> *¼ ripe pineapple, scrubbed well or peeled if not organic*
> *1-inch piece ginger root, washed or peeled if not organic*

Cut the pineapple into pieces that will fit your juicer's feed tube. Juice the pineapple with the ginger. Stir the juice and pour into a glass. You can add 1 cup of water if it is too sweet. Serve at room temperature or chilled, as desired.

Makes about 8 ounces

Nature's Best Electrolyte Replacer

NUTRISIP: Why buy a pasteurized, nutrient-depleted electrolyte replacer when you can make your own organic, nutrient-rich electrolyte replacement drink? For all workouts and sports events that last longer than an hour, you'll want to prevent your electrolyte balance from getting too low. Drink one-half cup of electrolyte replacer every 20 minutes during an event or long workout.

> *2 medium oranges, peeled*
> *4 lemons, washed or peeled if not organic*
> *11½ limes, washed or peeled if not organic*
> *2 tablespoons honey*
> *Pinch of sea salt*
> *2 quarts cold water*

Cut the oranges, lemons, and limes into sections that will fit your juicer's feed tube. Juice them, and pour the juice into a large container. Add the honey, salt, and water; stir to combine. Chill.

Makes 2½ quarts

Hot Ginger-Lemon Tea

NUTRISIP: This tea is warming on a cold, wet day. It also is helpful for colds, sore throats, bronchitis, flu, and indigestion.

2-inch piece ginger root, washed
1/2 lemon, washed or peeled if not organic
2 cups water
1 tablespoon loose licorice tea (optional)
1 cinnamon stick, broken
4 to 5 whole cloves
Dash of ground nutmeg and ground cardamom

Juice the ginger with the lemon. Pour the ginger-lemon juice in a non-reactive small saucepan and add the water, licorice tea (as desired), cinnamon, cloves, nutmeg, and cardamom. Bring the mixture to a boil. Reduce the heat and simmer for 5 to 10 minutes. Strain the tea, pour into 2 mugs, and serve immediately.

Makes 2 servings

FIZZES

YOU CAN MAKE YOUR OWN pop (or fizzes, as I call them) with fruit juice and mineral water. If you are concerned about chemicals, artificial ingredients, and sugar, this is your healthiest choice. Sweetened soft drinks contain large quantities of sugar; a 12-ounce can of sugar-sweetened soda pop contains seven to eight teaspoons of refined sugar. Sugar-free drinks contain artificial sweeteners such as aspartame, which can adversely affect health. Reporting in the *Journal of the Advancement of Medicine,* researchers state that, according to the National Cancer Institute, there has been a significant increase in malignant brain cancers since 1985; this followed within two years of the licensing of aspartame in beverages. They also note a large number of aspartame-related seizures. Many diet soft drinks contain phosphates as well, which can interfere with calcium absorption.

Over the last three decades, soft drink consumption among children and teens has more than tripled. The prevalence of childhood obesity doubled in that same time period. There also has been a 300 percent increase in the consumption of non-citrus juices in that same time period among young children. Switching from sugar-sweetened or artificially sweetened and high-calorie drinks to 100 percent freshly made fruit juice with mineral water is highly recommended.

Berry Cool

NUTRISIP: Berries are a source of catechins, phytonutrients that show promise in supporting the immune system and lowering cholesterol.

> *½ Golden Delicious organic apple, washed*
> *1 cup blackberries or raspberries, rinsed*
> *½ to 1 cup unsweetened mineral water*

Cut the half apple in half and juice with the berries. Pour the juice into a glass and add the mineral water. Stir to combine and add ice, if desired, or serve chilled.

Makes 8 to 12 ounces

Sparkling Cranberry Apple

NUTRISIP: Researchers have found that those who consume the most apples have reduced tension and less sickness in general.

> *2 Golden Delicious organic apples, washed*
> *¼ cup fresh or frozen (thawed) cranberries, rinsed*
> *¼ lemon, washed or peeled if not organic*
> *½ cup unsweetened mineral water*

Cut the apples into sections that will fit your juicer's feed tube. With the juicer turned off, add the cranberries, followed by the apple, lemon, and plunger. Juice the fruits. Pour the juice into a glass and add the mineral water. Stir to combine and add ice, as desired, or serve chilled.

Makes 10 to 12 ounces

Sparkling Strawberry

NUTRISIP: A source of the phytonutrients P-coumaric acid and chlorogenic acid, strawberries block the production of cancer-causing nitrosamines.

> *½ Golden Delicious organic apple, washed*
> *5 to 7 organic strawberries, washed*
> *¼ lemon, washed or peeled if not organic*
> *½ cup unsweetened mineral water*

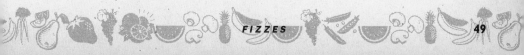

Halve the half apple; juice it with the strawberries and lemon. Pour the juice into a glass, add the mineral water, stir to combine, and add ice or serve chilled.

Makes 8 to 10 ounces

Ginger Ale Plus

NUTRISIP: Ginger offers a plant chemical called gingerol, which is a more powerful antioxidant than vitamin E.

2 Golden Delicious organic apples, washed
2-inch piece ginger root, washed
$1/2$ to 1 cup unsweetened mineral water

Cut the apples to fit into your juicer's feed tube. Juice with the ginger. Pour into a glass, add the mineral water, stir to combine, and add ice or serve chilled.

Makes 10 to 14 ounces

Skinny Sip

NUTRISIP: With only five calories, this is an ideal low-calorie, vitamin C–rich thirst quencher.

$1/2$ lemon, washed or peeled if not organic
1 cup unsweetened mineral water

Juice the lemon and pour the juice into a glass. Add the mineral water and stir to combine. Add ice, as desired, or serve chilled.

Makes about 8 ounces

Limeade Sparkler

NUTRISIP: Limes and other citrus fruits offer *triterpenoids*. Sound like something you'd find in your shampoo? Actually, they are phytonutrients that prevent dental decay and bind to estrogens, thus helping prevent breast cancer.

1 Golden Delicious organic apple, washed
1/2 lime, washed or peeled if not organic
1 cup unsweetened mineral water

Cut the apple into sections that will fit your juicer's feed tube. Juice them with the lime. Pour the juice into a glass and add the mineral water. Stir to combine and pour into a glass. Add ice, as desired, or serve chilled.

Makes about 10 ounces

Island Breeze

NUTRISIP: Limonoids are phytonutrients found in citrus fruits; they help protect the body from cancer-causing agents.

1 orange, peeled
2-inch chunk of pineapple, scrubbed well or peeled if not organic
1 kiwifruit, washed or peeled if not organic
1/2 cup unsweetened mineral water

Cut the orange and pineapple into pieces that will fit your juicer's feed tube. Cut the kiwi in half. Juice the orange, pineapple, and kiwi. Pour the juice into a glass. Add the mineral water and stir to combine. Add ice, as desired, or serve chilled.

Makes 10 to 12 ounces

Orange-Apple Cooler

NUTRISIP: Citrus fruits are sources of the phytonutrients called coumarins, which help prevent blood clotting.

2 Golden Delicious organic apples, washed
1 orange, peeled
4 mint sprigs, rinsed
1/4 lemon, washed or peeled if not organic
1 cup unsweetened mineral water

Cut the apples and the orange into pieces that will fit your juicer's feed tube. Bunch up the mint and juice it with the apples, orange, and lemon. Pour the juice into 2 glasses and add half of the mineral water to each. Stir to combine and add ice, as desired, or serve chilled.

Makes 16 ounces

Grapefruit-Orange Spritzer

NUTRISIP: Red grapefruit offers lycopene, a phytonutrient that is a powerful antioxidant that helps the body resist cancer.

½ red grapefruit, peeled
½ orange, peeled
½ cup unsweetened mineral water

Cut the grapefruit and orange into sections and juice them. Pour the juice into a glass and add the mineral water. Stir to combine and add ice, as desired, or serve chilled.

Makes about 8 ounces

Cherry Fizz

NUTRISIP: The flavonoids in cherries have been shown to help prevent periodontal disease.

½ organic apple (any variety), washed
1 cup organic cherries, washed and pitted
½ cup unsweetened mineral water

Cut the half apple in half and juice it with the cherries. Pour the juice into a glass and add the mineral water. Stir to combine and add ice, as desired, or serve chilled.

Makes 8 to 10 ounces

Minty Melon Refresher

NUTRISIP: Mint contains the phytonutrient monoterpene, which has antioxidant properties and also facilitates protective enzyme activity.

¼ ripe honeydew melon, washed or peeled if not organic
3 to 4 mint sprigs, rinsed
½ cup unsweetened mineral water

Cut the melon into pieces that will fit your juicer's feed tube. Bunch up the mint and juice it with the melon. Pour the juice into a glass and add the mineral water. Stir to combine and add ice, as desired, or serve chilled.

Makes 8 to 10 ounces

SMOOTHIES

SMOOTHIE BARS ARE POPPING UP all over the country. Smoothies are popular because they are delicious and healthy. By making smoothies at home, you can choose the most nutritious ingredients. You can also add nutrition boosters such as extra vitamin C, ginseng, bee pollen, protein powder, or fiber for a lot less money than you would spend for the same ingredients at a smoothie bar.

A fresh-fruit smoothie is a great breakfast option for the whole family. You can pack a smoothie with nutrients and healthful ingredients that can boost energy levels, improve brainpower, and strengthen immune functions. For example, mangos, apricots, cantaloupes, papayas, nectarines, prunes, carrots, and peaches are all rich sources of beta carotene, an important antioxidant for strengthening the immune system. As far back as 1931, scientists discovered that schoolchildren who had diets rich in carotenes (measured by blood levels) missed the least number of school days due to illness.

A smoothie makes a great meal replacement for breakfast, lunch, or dinner if you are trying to lose a few pounds. Many smoothies are under 300 calories, and some are just over 100 calories, yet they are yummy and filling.

Here's another idea: Smoothies make great desserts, especially when you freeze them. Frozen smoothies are much more healthful than ice cream or frozen yogurt. I discovered just how good they could be when my husband, who is the official taste tester for all my recipes, said he couldn't possibly look at another smoothie. No wonder! I had given him about six that day. Not wanting to waste the rest of my creations, I froze them. They were delicious! John heartily approved, and Freezes (see page 63) were born.

Tropical Sunrise

NUTRISIP: Pineapple contains bromelain—a protein-digesting enzyme that helps break down animal and plant proteins and improves digestion.

3-inch chunk of pineapple, scrubbed well or peeled if not organic
1 medium banana, peeled
½ medium papaya, peeled and seeded
½ cup plain or vanilla soy milk (or plain yogurt or milk)
¼ teaspoon pure vanilla extract
6 ice cubes

Cut the pineapple into pieces that will fit your juicer's feed tube and juice it. Pour the juice into a blender and add the banana, papaya, soy milk, vanilla, and ice cubes. Blend the mixture until smooth. Pour it into 2 glasses and serve.

Makes about 16 ounces

Rise 'n' Shake

NUTRISIP: Oranges are a good source of vitamin C and bioflavonoids (phytonutrients), which are found mainly in the white pithy part of the orange. Vitamin C and bioflavonoids work together to strengthen blood vessel walls.

2 medium oranges, peeled
1 medium banana, peeled
½ cup nonfat plain yogurt or plain soy milk
1 teaspoon pure vanilla extract
6 ice cubes
1 tablespoon protein powder (optional)

Cut the oranges into sections and juice them. Pour the juice into a blender and add the banana, yogurt, vanilla, ice cubes, and protein powder, as desired. Blend the mixture until smooth. Pour it into a glass and serve.

Makes 8 to 10 ounces

The Champ

NUTRISIP: Spinach and parsley contain vitamin C and iron, which nature packed perfectly in these foods because vitamin C enhances the absorption of iron. For those who are fatigued due to low iron supplies, this is a champion smoothie for boosting energy levels.

½ Golden or Red Delicious organic apple, washed
1 handful organic spinach with stems, washed
4 parsley sprigs, washed
1 medium banana, peeled
1 tablespoon tahini (sesame paste)
6 ice cubes

Cut the half apple in half and bunch up the spinach and parsley. Tuck them in the feed tube first, then the apple, and juice them. Pour the juice into a blender and add the banana, tahini, and ice. Blend the mixture until smooth. Pour it into 1 or 2 glasses and serve.

Makes about 16 ounces

Muscle Power Plus

NUTRISIP: Bananas, tofu, and peanuts are good sources of potassium. You may be surprised to learn that, ounce for ounce, peanuts have more potassium than bananas. Potassium is one of the electrolytes—a mineral salt that conducts electricity when dissolved in water. Muscle weakness, problems with muscle contraction, and fatigue can be symptoms of potassium deficiency.

½ Golden Delicious organic apple, washed
1 medium banana, peeled
1 tablespoon peanut butter (creamy or crunchy)
½ cup silken tofu or nonfat plain yogurt
6 ice cubes

Cut the apple into sections that will fit your juicer's feed tube and juice it. Pour the apple juice into a blender and add the banana, peanut butter, tofu

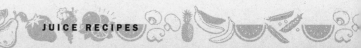

or yogurt, and ice cubes. Blend the mixture until smooth. Pour it into 1 or 2 glasses and serve.

Makes about 16 ounces

Bone Power Plus

NUTRISIP: Ounce for ounce, tofu has more calcium and magnesium than yogurt or milk—two minerals that work together to build healthy bones. Deep blue-red berries, such as blueberries, blackberries, and raspberries, are rich in anthocyanidins and proanthocyanidins—flavonoids that stabilize collagen structures. This is significant because collagen is the major protein structure of bone. All these ingredients together make an excellent bone-strengthening smoothie.

½ Golden or Red Delicious organic apple, washed
1 cup blueberries, blackberries, or raspberries, washed
¼ lemon, washed or peeled if not organic
1 banana, peeled
½ cup silken tofu (nonfat plain yogurt can be substituted)
6 ice cubes

Cut the apple into sections that will fit your juicer's feed tube. Juice the apple with the berries and lemon. Pour the juice into a blender and add the banana, tofu or yogurt, and ice cubes. Blend the mixture until smooth. Pour it into 1 or 2 glasses and serve.

Makes about 16 ounces

Mango Mania

NUTRISIP: Mango has been used as a folk remedy to improve circulation.

2 kiwifruits, washed or peeled if not organic
1 ripe mango, peeled
1 ripe banana, peeled
6 ice cubes

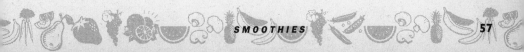

Cut the kiwis in half and juice. Pour the juice into a blender. Cut the mango in pieces from the stone and add them to the blender with the banana and ice cubes. Blend the mixture until smooth. Pour it into 2 glasses and serve.

Makes about 20 ounces

Cherries Jubilation

NUTRISIP: Cherries contain flavonoids that have the ability to support collagen structure and prevent collagen destruction. Collagen is responsible for a number of functions, one of which is giving skin its youthful appearance.

1 cup organic cherries, washed and pitted
½ cup nonfat plain yogurt
½ teaspoon pure vanilla extract
½ teaspoon honey
6 ice cubes

Juice the cherries and pour the juice into a blender. Add the yogurt, vanilla, honey, and ice cubes. Blend the mixture until smooth. Pour it into 1 or 2 glasses and serve.

Makes about 16 ounces

Berry Smooth

NUTRISIP: Cashews are one of the richest sources of magnesium. A number of studies have found that people with a high magnesium intake have healthier blood pressure levels.

2 large Golden Delicious organic apples, washed
1 cup berries (raspberries, blackberries, or blueberries)
⅓ cup raw cashews
½ teaspoon pure vanilla extract
6 ice cubes

Cut the apples into sections that will fit your juicer's feed tube. Juice the apples and berries. Pour the juice into a blender and add the cashews, vanilla, and ice cubes; blend the mixture until smooth. Pour it into 1 or 2 glasses and serve.

Makes about 16 ounces

Spicy Peaches 'n' Cream

NUTRISIP: Peach juice is a traditional remedy for digestion. Try this smoothie for a tasty treat as well as for intestinal relief after a heavy meal. Since peaches are available only from June through September, you may choose to substitute frozen peaches at other times of the year. In this case, add the peaches (thawed) to the blender. If you can't find frozen peaches (they are healthier than canned), choose peaches canned in their own juice rather than syrup.

> 2 ripe peaches, washed (peeled if not organic), stones removed
> $\frac{1}{2}$ Golden or Red Delicious organic apple, washed
> 2-inch piece ginger root, washed
> $\frac{1}{2}$ cup nonfat plain yogurt (silken tofu may be substituted)
> 1 teaspoon pure vanilla extract
> 1 to 2 teaspoons honey
> $\frac{1}{2}$ teaspoon ground cinnamon
> 6 ice cubes

Cut the peaches and apple into sections that will fit your juicer's feed tube. Juice the peaches, apple, and ginger; pour the juice into a blender. Add the yogurt or tofu, vanilla, honey, cinnamon, and ice cubes. Blend the mixture until smooth. Pour it into a glass and serve.

Makes 12 to 14 ounces

Strawberry-Almond Surprise

NUTRISIP: In a recent study it was found that strawberries and spinach had the highest antioxidant activity of 40 common fruits and vegetables.

1 cup organic strawberries, washed
1 ripe medium banana, peeled
1/2 cup blanched almonds
1/2 cup plain or vanilla soy milk (dairy milk can be substituted)
1/2 teaspoon pure vanilla extract
2 to 3 drops pure almond extract (optional)
6 ice cubes

Juice the strawberries and pour the juice in a blender. Add the banana, almonds, milk, vanilla, almond extract (if using), and ice cubes. Blend the mixture until smooth. Pour it into 1 or 2 glasses.

Makes about 16 ounces

Tropical Treat

NUTRISIP: Papaya is a source of carotenoids—those marvelous antioxidants that keep us healthy.

1 medium orange, peeled
1/4 lime, washed or peeled if not organic
1/2 ripe medium Hawaiian papaya, or 1/4 medium Mexican papaya,
   seeds removed, peeled
1 ripe medium banana, peeled
6 ice cubes

Cut the orange into sections that will fit your juicer's feed tube. Juice the orange with the lime. Pour the juice into a blender. Add the papaya, banana, and ice. Blend the mixture until smooth. Pour it into 2 or 3 glasses and serve.

Makes about 24 ounces

Lemon Lite

NUTRISIP: Refreshing on a summer day, lemons contain citrus flavonoids—
antioxidants that increase intracellular levels of vitamin C.

1 medium Golden Delicious organic apple, washed
½ lemon, washed or peeled if not organic
1 banana, peeled
½ cup nonfat plain yogurt
6 to 7 ice cubes

Cut the apple into sections that will fit your juicer's feed tube. Juice the
apple with the lemon and pour the juice into a blender. Add the banana,
yogurt, and ice cubes. Blend the mixture until smooth. Pour it into 1 or 2
glasses and serve.

Makes about 16 ounces

Spicy Coconut Delight

NUTRISIP: Coconut contains manganese, a mineral that contributes to
healthy skin, hair, and nails. In a number of human studies where partici-
pants were given a manganese-deficient diet, abnormalities developed,
including skin rashes, loss of hair color, and reduced growth of hair and
nails.

2-inch chunk of pineapple, scrubbed well or peeled if not organic
2-inch piece ginger root, washed
1 banana, peeled
½ cup low-fat coconut milk (soy milk can be substituted)
6 ice cubes

Cut the pineapple into pieces that will fit your juicer's feed tube. Juice the
pineapple with the ginger. Pour the juice into a blender. Add the banana,
coconut milk or soy milk, and ice cubes. Blend the mixture until smooth.
Pour it into 1 or 2 glasses.

Makes about 16 ounces

Cherie's Quick-Energy Soup

NUTRISIP: Though people sometimes think of avocado as high in fat and therefore to be avoided, it does not contain saturated fat—the fats in avocado are healthy. In one study, 15 females were given either a diet high in monounsaturated fatty acids enriched with avocado, or a high-complex-carbohydrate diet for three weeks, after which the other diet was given. Both diets reduced cholesterol, compared to the baseline, but the avocado-enriched diet was more effective, showing an 8.2 percent reduction in cholesterol versus a 4.9 percent reduction on the complex carbohydrate diet.

1¼ cups fresh carrot juice (7 to 8 medium carrots)
1 avocado, peeled, seed removed
½ teaspoon ground cumin

Place the carrot juice, avocado, and cumin in a blender and puree until smooth. Chill until ready to serve. Pour the mixture into a bowl and add any of the following: chopped basil, grated zucchini, carrot, beet, or fresh corn cut from the cob.

Makes 14 to 16 ounces

FREEZES

FRUIT SORBETS ARE A HEALTHFUL ALTERNATIVE to ice cream and frozen yogurt. You can make your own frozen desserts that are refined-sugar-free, fat-reduced or fat-free, and free of additives, dyes, and preservatives. There are no lists of names you can't pronounce in these desserts—just pure ingredients that you choose. The taste of fruit is refreshingly delicious. In addition, you will know you are giving yourself and your loved ones a dessert that is truly good for everyone.

On a hot summer day, almost nothing can replace a cool, delicious Popsicle. But "frozen pops" don't have to be unhealthy to be delicious. You can make your own by freezing your favorite fruit juice combinations in either plastic pop molds or ice cube trays; stir in some of the fruit pulp with the juice to give them texture, as desired.

Commercial Popsicles usually have added sugars, dyes, preservatives, and other additives. They also are more expensive than the homemade version. Get creative with your own combinations—try strawberry-kiwi, watermelon, grape-apple, or lemonade. You can also make creamy frozen pops by adding soy milk, dairy milk, or yogurt to fruit juice. How about a creamy orange, strawberry, or peach Creamsicle (see page 67)?

Orange Sorbet

NUTRISIP: Oranges contain carotenoids, antioxidants that protect against cancer and that may help reduce accumulation of arterial plaque.

3 medium oranges, peeled
1/2 cup vanilla soy milk
1 teaspoon pure vanilla extract

Cut the oranges into sections that will fit your juicer's feed tube. Juice the oranges (you should have about 1½ cups of juice).

In a medium bowl, combine the juice, soy milk, and vanilla, mixing well. Pour the mixture into a shallow metal or plastic dish, cover, and freeze until solid, 3 to 4 hours.

Using a metal spatula, break the frozen sorbet into chunks and place them in a food processor; blend until smooth and creamy. Stop the food processor occasionally to scrape down the sides and stir the sorbet. Serve immediately, or freeze in a covered container until ready to serve.

Makes 4 servings

Strawberry Sorbet

NUTRISIP: Strawberries are a source of ellagic acid, a phytonutrient that has cancer-prevention effects.

1 Golden Delicious organic apple, washed
1 ripe organic pear, washed
1 cup organic strawberries with caps, washed
⅓ cup soy milk
2 tablespoons pure vanilla extract

Cut the apple and pear into pieces that will fit your juicer's feed tube. Juice the strawberries first; reserve all the juice and pulp. Juice the apple and pear.

In a medium bowl, combine the strawberry juice and pulp, apple-pear juice, soy milk, and vanilla, mixing well. Pour the mixture into a shallow metal or plastic container, cover, and freeze until solid, 3 to 4 hours.

Using a metal spatula, break the frozen sorbet into chunks and place them in a food processor; blend until smooth and creamy. Stop the food processor occasionally to scrape down the sides and stir the sorbet. Serve immediately, or freeze in a covered container until ready to serve.

Makes 4 servings

Pineapple Sorbet

NUTRISIP: Pineapple is a source of calcium and magnesium. Though these minerals are not particularly high in pineapple (the calcium is about one-tenth of that found in milk), it is one more source for these important minerals that keep bones strong.

1 small ripe pineapple, scrubbed well or peeled if not organic
2 tablespoons honey
2 teaspoons pure vanilla extract

Cut the pineapple into pieces that will fit your juicer's feed tube. Juice the pineapple and reserve 2 cups of the juice and 1 cup of the pulp.

In a medium bowl, combine the pineapple juice, pulp, honey, and vanilla, mixing well. Pour the mixture into a shallow metal or plastic dish, cover, and freeze until solid, 3 to 4 hours.

Using a metal spatula, break the frozen sorbet into chunks and place them in a food processor; blend until smooth and creamy. Stop the food processor occasionally to scrape down the sides and stir the sorbet. Serve immediately, or return to the freezer in a covered container until ready to serve.

Makes 4 servings

Lemon Sorbet

NUTRISIP: For years English ships were required to carry enough lemon or lime juice for each sailor to have an ounce per day after the tenth day at sea to prevent scurvy. That's why English sailors were nicknamed "limeys."

5 medium Golden or Red Delicious organic apples, washed
1 lemon, washed or peeled if not organic
3 tablespoons honey

Cut the apples into sections that will fit your juicer's feed tube. Cut the lemon in half and juice it with the apples.

In a medium bowl, combine the apple-lemon juice and honey; mix well. Pour the mixture into a shallow metal or plastic dish, cover, and freeze until solid, 3 to 4 hours.

Using a metal spatula, break the frozen sorbet into chunks and place them in a food processor; blend until smooth and creamy. Stop the food processor occasionally to scrape down the sides and stir the sorbet. Serve immediately, or freeze in a covered container until ready to serve.

Makes 4 servings

Cantaloupe Sorbet

NUTRISIP: Cantaloupe is rich in beta carotene; this carotene strengthens the immune system.

> *1 (organic if Mexican) cantaloupe, washed or peeled if not organic*
> *1 cup fresh mint, rinsed*
> *2 tablespoons honey*

Cut the cantaloupe into pieces. Bunch up the mint and juice it with the cantaloupe. Pour the cantaloupe-mint juice into a medium bowl and add the honey, mixing well. Pour the mixture into a shallow metal or plastic dish, cover, and freeze until solid, 3 to 4 hours.

Using a metal spatula, break the frozen sorbet into chunks and place them in a food processor; blend until smooth and creamy. Stop the food processor occasionally to scrape down the sides and stir the sorbet. Serve immediately, or freeze in a covered container until ready to serve.

Makes 4 servings

Lemon-Mint Sorbet

NUTRISIP: Mint contains azulene, found in the oil, which has anti-inflammatory effects.

> *1 large lemon, washed or peeled if not organic*
> *6 large mint sprigs, rinsed*
> *1 tablespoon honey*
> *1 cup water*
> *1 egg white, beaten until stiff*

Cut the lemon in half; bunch up the mint, and juice the mint with the lemon. Set the juice aside.

Boil the water and honey until dissolved. Remove from the heat and add the lemon-mint juice; let stand until cool.

Pour the mixture into a metal or plastic dish, cover, and freeze until half frozen (1½ to 2 hours).

Fold in the beaten egg white and refreeze for 1½ to 2 hours.

Using a metal spatula, break the frozen sorbet into chunks and place them in a food processor; blend until smooth and creamy. Stop the food processor occasionally to scrape down the sides and stir the sorbet. Serve immediately, or return to the freezer in a covered container until ready to serve.

Makes 4 servings

Orange, Strawberry, or Peach Creamsicles

NUTRISIP: Phenolic acids are plant chemicals that are found in citrus fruits and berries. They help the body resist cancer by inhibiting nitrosamine formation.

> 2 medium oranges, peeled; or
>> 1 pint organic strawberries with caps, washed; or
>> 1½ pounds ripe organic peaches, washed (need 1 cup of juice)
> 1 Golden Delicious organic apple, washed (need ½ cup of juice)
> 1 teaspoon honey
> ½ teaspoon pure vanilla extract
> 2 tablespoons soy milk, dairy milk, or nonfat plain yogurt

Cut the oranges or peaches into pieces that will fit your juicer's feed tube. Juice the oranges, strawberries, or peaches with the apple. Pour the juice into a blender, add the honey, vanilla, and milk or yogurt; blend until smooth. Pour the mixture into individual plastic pop molds or ice cube trays and freeze for 2 to 3 hours.

Makes about 12 ounces

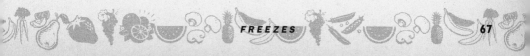

II

JUICING FOR VIBRANT GOOD LOOKS

When my grandmother told me that beauty was more than skin deep, I knew she was talking about integrity, generosity, and love. Biologically, beauty is more than skin deep as well; it begins in the organs of elimination and digestion, right down in the cells. In science it comes down to biochemistry. And it all starts with what you put in your mouth.

I still remember a story told by Gayelord Hauser (a leading nutritionist and beauty expert in the '70s) about a young woman he met at a party. She was surrounded by scores of beautiful people—perfect features, right makeup, gorgeous clothes. She didn't have perfect features and was dressed simply, but she stood out from everyone else because she looked so incredibly healthy—and that was what made her the most beautiful woman in the room.

You and I may not have the most beautiful faces in the world, but we all have an opportunity to exude the vibrant good looks of health. That beauty is uniquely yours. Your beauty potential lies in what you eat and drink, breathe, and think. So watch out for beauty thieves— anything that robs your body of its good-looks potential.

Come along with me through the pages of Juicing for Vibrant Good Looks and I'll teach you how to look and feel your best through the miracle power of "live food in a glass."

LOOK YOUNGER

To SLOW AGING AND START looking younger, it is important to know what causes aging. Along with wear and tear and aging DNA and molecules, it is generally accepted that free-radical damage contributes greatly to the aging process. Free radicals are highly reactive molecules that lack an electron. They attack cells to steal an electron to make them stable and damage cells in the process. The damaged cells then become free radicals, setting in motion a chain reaction. Free-radical damage contributes to wrinkles, sagging skin, loss of muscle tone, age spots, and the onset of age-related diseases. Cross-linking of proteins (collagen and elastin) to other molecules also can occur, making each cell less flexible and adaptable; we know this process through wrinkles and dry and leathery skin.

Aging is understood to be a weakening and decline of the body, which begins as soon as physical growth stops. From that moment on our powers decline gradually throughout adulthood, unless lifestyle factors accelerate or retard the process.

DIETARY RECOMMENDATIONS

Looking younger begins with what you eat. The following tips will help you look and feel better.

1. *Consume more raw fruits and vegetables and fresh juices.* How do we protect ourselves from free radicals? Easy. Mother Nature has provided us with a group of compounds known as antioxidants. These vitamins, minerals, enzymes, and phytonutrients bind to free radicals and carry them out of your body. Fruits and vegetables and fresh juices are loaded with antioxidants. (For more information on the benefits of raw food, see Basic Guidelines for the Vibrant Health Diet, page 174.)

2. *Use periodic juice fasting.*   Whether you choose to juice-fast one day a week or two to three days a month, you can watch the lines disappear and your vitality increase. Research suggests that one way to slow down the rate of cross-linkage (wrinkling and loss of elasticity) is to eat sparingly and to fast occasionally. Juice fasting gives your body a rest from the taxing digestive processes because there is no solid food to digest. Raw juices are loaded with plant enzymes that spare your organs the work of making enzymes to digest food. This allows your body time to concentrate on repair and rejuvenation. Fresh juices provide an abundance of nutrients that heal and restore the body. They also contain a special energy derived from the sun during photosynthesis, which cooking virtually destroys. I often juice-fast one day a week when I'm home, and I take one or two weeks a year to juice-fast at a health institute or spa. I always return home looking younger, people say, and definitely feeling renewed. (For more information, see Juice Fasting, page 160.)

3. *Decrease sugar consumption.*   Research data implies that higher amounts of sucrose may fuel the aging process. Animal studies indicate that larger amounts of sucrose in the diet of rodents reduces their life span.

4. *Reduce calories.*   Several studies point to the fact that eating less food may contribute to longevity—certainly to a trimmer body. If you get adequate amounts of protein, fat, carbohydrates, vitamins, minerals, phytonutrients, and enzymes while eating fewer calories, it may be possible to slow aging considerably. This was shown in studies with rodents and monkeys. Decreasing calories by 30 percent for 200 monkeys reduced metabolic changes that are markers for aging.

NUTRIENT RECOMMENDATIONS

- *Carotenes.* Beta carotene and lycopene are among nature's most potent antioxidants. There is evidence that the more carotenes present in tissues, the longer the life span. Best juice sources: dandelion greens, carrots, kale, parsley, spinach, beet greens, watercress, mangos, cantaloupes, and apricots.

- *Vitamin C.* Vitamin C is an antioxidant that has protective effects that keep cells from free-radical damage. One study showed that subjects 50 years old or more who consumed the greatest amount of vitamin C were clinically similar to the 40-year-olds who were consuming the least amount of vitamin C. Best juice sources: kale, parsley, broccoli, Brussels sprouts, watercress, strawberries, papayas, spinach, oranges, lemons, and grapefruit.

- *Vitamin E.* This is a powerful antioxidant. Studies have shown there is an increased need for vitamin E, especially when oxidative stress is increased and at higher altitudes. Vitamin E can help prevent lipid peroxidation (age spots). Best juice sources: spinach, asparagus, carrots, and tomatoes.

- *Selenium.* This is another key antioxidant. In one study with over 100 people, aging was associated with a decrease in selenium status. Best juice sources: turnips, garlic, oranges, and grapes.

- *Enzymes.* The most powerful free-radical-scavenging enzymes are superoxide dismutase (SOD), catalase, and glutathione peroxidase. Best juice sources: all fruits and vegetables.

- *Phytonutrients.* Many phytonutrients are antioxidants. Carotenoids, found in parsley, carrots, cantaloupes, apricots, spinach, kale, turnip greens, and citrus fruits, are significant factors in determining maximum life span (MLS). Flavonoids, found in parsley, carrots, citrus fruits, cabbage, cucumbers, tomatoes, and berries, have a positive effect on collagen, which maintains "ground substance." Ground substance holds tissues together and supports skin structure. In particular, the flavonoids—proanthocyanidins and PCOs (procyanidolic oligomers)—found in berries and grapes, offer much greater antioxidant activity than vitamins C and E; they significantly delay the onset of lipid peroxidation (age spots) and bind to free iron molecules, thus preventing iron-induced lipid peroxidation.

- *HCl betaine.* As we age, the body produces less and less hydrochloric acid (stomach acid). Hydrochloric acid (HCl) kills bacteria in the stomach and breaks down food as part of the digestive process. Supplemental HCl betaine aids digestion and may be beneficial in slowing aging. (It is sold at most health food stores.)

- *Melatonin.* This free-radical-scavenging antioxidant is a hormone secreted by the pineal gland. Studies show that melatonin can retard the rate of aging and the time of onset of age-related diseases. (It is available at most health food stores.)

JUICE RECOMMENDATIONS

Specific juice recommendations: *Watermelon, celery, carrot, and parsley.*

The following recipes are suggestions for juice combinations using the fruits and vegetables highest in the nutrients recommended for antiaging.

1. Sources of carotenes: The Morning Energizer (page 16) and Santa Fe Salsa Cocktail (page 19)

2. Sources of vitamin C: Morning Sunrise (page 39) and Rise 'n' Shake smoothie (page 55)

3. Sources of selenium: Morning Express (page 20) and The Immune Builder (page 31)

4. Sources of vitamin E: Popeye's Power (page 21) and Spring Tonic (page 33)

5. Sources of carotenoids and flavonoids: Strawberry-Cantaloupe Cocktail (page 38) and Beautiful Hair, Skin, and Nails Solution (page 84)

6. Sources of the anthocyanidins and proanthocyanidins (flavonoids found in grapes, particularly the seeds, and berries): Antiaging Solution (page 39) and Grape Expectations (page 40)

PREVENT or CORRECT AGE SPOTS

AGE SPOTS, ALSO KNOWN AS liver spots, are flat brown areas that appear on the skin as it ages. They result from lipofuscin accumulation, a by-product of lipid peroxidation (damage to fat). Fats and cholesterol, also known as lipids, are particularly susceptible to free-radical damage. When lipids are damaged, they form by-products known as lipid peroxides and cholesterol epoxides. These waste by-products of fat damage occur internally as well as externally. Externally, we can see the skin color change to brown-gold or dark brown. But this free-radical damage is occurring internally as well, including in the liver cells and brain cells. Though age spots are thought to be harmless, they are actually signals that cells are filled with accumulated waste and are being destroyed. Age spots can be removed, which can improve appearance, but this does nothing to correct the free-radical damage occurring inside the body.

Age spots can be caused by poor diet, nutrient deficiencies, poor liver function, rancid oil ingestion, lack of exercise, cigarette smoke, stress, and excess sun exposure. High altitudes and exposure to ultraviolet light can accelerate the process. Age spots reflect cumulative skin damage, so the use of sunscreen early in life will help prevent photoaging.

DIETARY RECOMMENDATIONS

Nutritional intervention has been shown to aid in the reduction of lipofuscin deposits. Dietary antioxidants protect skin cells from free-radical destruction. If a free radical reacts with an antioxidant rather than with a cell membrane, cell damage can be prevented. Antioxidants such as vitamins C and E, selenium, coenzyme Q10, and such phytonutrients as the citrus flavonoids and carotenoids will inhibit damage that results in lipofuscin deposits. Antioxidant nutrients are found in high concentration in wheatgrass juice and barley grass juice, sprouts, and leafy dark green vegetables. Powerful free-radical protection is provided by the antioxidant combination of beta carotene and superoxide dismutase, available in wheatgrass juice.

1. *Eat your vegetables and fruits and drink freshly made juices.* Raw fruits and vegetables are loaded with antioxidants and other important nutrients that protect your cells from damage. Once vegetables and fruits are cooked, many of the antioxidants are destroyed. Raw fruits and vegetables also help detoxify the body, which means getting rid of accumulated wastes like lipofuscin. Beets are especially cleansing for the liver. For more information, see Basic Guidelines for the Vibrant Health Diet, page 174.

2. *Use periodic juice fasting.* One to three days of juice fasting will help cleanse your body at the cellular level. As you abstain from eating solid food, which requires considerable work for digestion, your body can focus on cleanup and repair. Juices are already broken down from insoluble fiber, so very little digestive work is required. A juice fast is a vacation for your digestive system and an opportunity for your body to clean out the wastes that have accumulated, including the brown slime called lipofuscin. Raw juices provide scores of helpers in the form of antioxidants that scavenge free radicals, thus preventing further damage to cells. They also offer other nutrients that repair and restore cells, soluble fibers that act as "internal brooms," and nutrient-rich water that flushes out accumulated wastes. For more information, see Juice Fasting, page 160. To get rid of age spots, it is especially helpful to cleanse the liver—see The Liver Cleanse, page 167.

3. *Avoid rancid oils.* This will help to prevent age spots. The destruction of cooking oil occurs when a bottle is opened and the oil is exposed to air. Oils always should be refrigerated once they are opened. Olive oil and canola oil, which are monounsaturated fats, undergo less oxidation than polyunsaturated oils. Olive oil contains vitamin E and is rich in antioxidant phenolic compounds. Unless an oil is unrefined, the high temperatures used in the hydrogenation process create trans-fatty acids (toxic fats). Margarine and shortening should be avoided because they are hydrogenated.

NUTRIENT RECOMMENDATIONS

- *Carotenes* such as beta carotene and lycopene are powerful antioxidants. They help protect the skin from ultraviolet light damage. Best juice sources: dandelion greens, carrots, kale, parsley, spinach, beet greens, watercress, mangoes, cantaloupes, and apricots.

- *Retinoic acid,* a vitamin A derivative used topically, has been shown to reverse age spots. Studies also show that vitamin A application improves skin elasticity and thickness. Vitamin A and provitamin A (carotenes) provide powerful antioxidant protection for cells. Best juice sources: carrots, kale, parsley, spinach, beet greens, watercress, mangos, bell peppers, squash, cantaloupes, and apricots.

- *Selenium* prevents cellular lipids from undergoing oxidation, the destruction that leads to age spots. Best juice sources: chard, turnips, garlic, oranges, and grapes.

- *Vitamin C* is a water-soluble antioxidant that scavenges free radicals and regenerates reduced vitamin E. It can help decrease the oxidative destruction associated with age spots. Best juice sources: bell peppers, kale, parsley, broccoli, Brussels sprouts, watercress, cauliflower, cabbage, strawberries, papayas, spinach, citrus fruits, mangos, and asparagus.

- *Flavonoids* work synergistically with Vitamin C to scavenge free radicals. Best juice sources: grapes, prunes, citrus fruits, cherries, plums, apricots, papayas, cantaloupes, parsley, cabbage, bell peppers, tomatoes, and broccoli.

- *Vitamin E* is a lipophilic antioxidant, which means it inhibits the peroxidation of lipids by quenching oxygen-free radicals. Research has shown that greater accumulation of lipofuscin has occurred during states of vitamin E deficiency. On a personal note, about three years prior to the time of this writing, we moved to Santa Fe, New Mexico, an elevation of 7,000 feet above sea level. Within months I noticed several small brown sun spots appearing on my hands. I couldn't figure out why these were occurring until I read research indicating that lipid peroxidation is accelerated at high elevations. I increased my vitamin E supplementation and was more careful about sun exposure. I didn't get any more spots, and the ones I had began to fade. Vitamin E, at 200 mg two times a day, has been shown to inhibit lipid peroxidation. Best juice sources: spinach, asparagus, carrots, and tomatoes.

JUICE RECOMMENDATIONS

Beets and *dandelion leaves* are good sources of liver-cleansing properties. Try The Morning Energizer (page 16) and Liver Life Cocktail (page 33).

The following recipes are suggested for juice combinations using the fruits and vegetables highest in the nutrients recommended to prevent and reverse age spots.

1. Sources of vitamin C and citrus flavonoids: Morning Express (page 20), Popeye's Power (page 21), Beautiful Bone Solution (page 25), and Morning Sunrise (page 39)

2. Sources of vitamin E: Spicy Tomato on Ice (page 19), The Colon Cleanser (page 26), and Spring Tonic (page 33)

3. Sources of selenium: The Immune Builder (page 31), Turnip Time (page 32), and Rise 'n' Shake smoothie (page 55)

4. Source of beta carotene and superoxide dismutase: Wheatgrass Light (page 21) and Pure Green Sprout Drink (page 22)

PREVENT or CORRECT CELLULITE

CELLULITE IS THE PRESENCE OF "orange peel" skin or what is called the "mattress" phenomenon, which is characterized by flattish protrusions and depressions of the skin. It is a cosmetic problem that commonly appears on the thighs and buttocks of women, indicating the adipose (fat cell) tissue has undergone degenerative changes. Though not related to obesity, excess weight can accentuate this condition.

Through ultrasonic analysis of the upper thigh and buttock tissue, a number of conclusions have been formed about cellulite. The lumps, bumps, pitting, and deformation is attributed to a deterioration of the dermal matrix (intercellular material) and capillary network, which leads to localized fluid retention. An increased concentration of glycosaminoglycans (polysaccharides linked to proteins that attract water) has been found in cellulite tissue, which leads to water retention. Also, there are changes in the "ground substance" (material that occupies intercellular spaces in fibrous connective tissue). In some cases it is possible that localized water retention results from inflammation, because inflammatory cells have been seen near the fat cells.

As we age, the layer just below the dermis (cornium layer) becomes thinner and looser, allowing more fat cells to migrate into the dermal layer (true skin). The connective tissue walls between fat cells become thinner, allowing the fat cells to enlarge. Toxins build up over time in the dermal layer, which is related to decreased lymphatic drainage, and consequently, waste and water collect around the fat cells. All this creates the *peau d'orange* (orange peel) appearance.

Correcting cellulite calls for a varied intervention. The goals are to (1) increase lymphatic drainage, (2) strengthen capillaries, (3) decrease glycosaminoglycan accumulation, (4) prevent degeneration of collagen and elastic fibers, and (5) decrease subcutaneous fat. Correction of cellulite may be accomplished through liposuction (if you have the money and the courage) or gradual weight loss, if that is needed (fast weight loss may worsen the condition due to rapid shrinking of fat cells), dietary changes, exercise, brush massage, professional massage, nutrient supplementation, topical and oral herbal prescriptions, and detoxification of the body. These approaches take dedication, but they work; and most important, they correct underlying problems that could lead to greater health challenges in years to come.

DIETARY AND LIFESTYLE RECOMMENDATIONS

1. *Eat a diet high in complex carbohydrates* and low in refined carbohydrates (sugar and white flour) and fat. A high-fiber diet helps remove cholesterol and fat from the body. For specific guidelines, see Basic Guidelines for the Vibrant Health Diet, page 174.

2. *Raw fruit and vegetable juices* are especially helpful in removing toxins, water, and waste. See the section "Drink Fresh Juice" under Basic Guidelines for the Vibrant Health Diet, page 174.

3. *Cleanse and detoxify your body.*   Cleansing the liver can be quite beneficial. Some researchers have found a correlation between poor liver function and cellulite. When you cleanse the liver it is advisable also to cleanse the kidneys. (See The Liver Cleanse, page 168, and The Kidney Cleanse Program, page 167.) It is believed that certain chemicals actually attract and hold water in the fat pockets associated with cellulite. A juice fast one day a week is terrific for helping to remove trapped toxins and water from the cellulite sites. Especially focus on juices that are natural diuretics (watermelon, cantaloupe, cucumber, parsley, lemon, asparagus, and kiwifruit). (See Juice Fasting, page 160.)

4. *Avoid sugar and all other refined carbohydrates, including white-flour products.*   Cakes, cookies, pies, ice cream, candy, chocolate, and other desserts are all great candidates for deposits into fat cells and offer nothing to build lean tissue.

5. *Avoid salt, alcohol, and soda pop.*   These substances interfere with efficient circulation of blood to the skin. Salt causes water retention. Soda pop is loaded with chemicals that can attract and hold water and chemicals, thus contributing to the problem. Alcohol acts like sugar in the body.

6. *Lose weight*—if needed. Studies show that women who are slim and athletic have the least amount of cellulite. Weight loss should be gradual, however, especially if you are over 40. Rapid weight loss in women this age can make the orange peel appearance more pronounced. (See Weight Loss, page 131.)

7. *Get regular exercise.* Exercise is a key to ridding your body of cellulite. As you lose fat and build lean tissue, you will notice encouraging improvements. (See the section on Exercise and Sports Endurance for more information on nutrition that will help with your get-up-and-go, page 123.)

8. *Massage and dry skin brushing* with a natural-bristle skin brush helps the skin. Purchase a long-handled, natural-bristle brush and brush up from your legs with long sweeping strokes. Regular skin brushing can greatly improve lymphatic drainage. If you can afford professional massage, this can also be very helpful in improving lymphatic drainage.

9. *Don't give up!* There is no quick fix to get rid of cellulite, other than surgery, which always poses some risks. The steps recommended here take time, but you should notice positive changes in several weeks to two months after starting this program. Stick with it. It will pay off. I know firsthand what dietary changes and exercise can accomplish. More than a decade ago, I had embarrassing cellulite. Now, it is almost completely gone.

NUTRIENT RECOMMENDATIONS

- *Bioflavonoids* work synergistically with vitamin C to strengthen capillaries. Best juice sources: grapes, prunes, citrus fruits, cherries, plums, apricots, papayas, cantaloupes, parsley, cabbage, bell peppers, tomatoes, and broccoli.

- *Vitamin C* has been shown to strengthen capillary walls. As these walls are strengthened, blood plasma has less chance of seeping through into spaces between cells, seepage which contributes to lumpy, bumpy skin. Best juice sources: bell peppers, kale, parsley, broccoli, watercress, cabbage, strawberries, papayas, spinach, citrus fruits, turnips, mangos, and asparagus.

- Vitamin E deficiency has been associated with capillary permeability. Best juice sources: spinach, asparagus, tomatoes, and carrots.

HERBAL RECOMMENDATIONS

- *Gotu kola (Cantella asiatica)* normalizes the metabolism of connective tissue by stimulating the manufacture of glycosaminoglycans (GAGs). This is a paradoxical effect in the treatment of cellulite, because an increased number of GAGs are found in cellulite tissue; however, clinically it has been found to be beneficial. The recommendation is 30 mg taken orally three times a day. (Look for this product at a health food store.)

- *Horse chestnut extract (Aesculus hippocastanum)* is an anti-inflammatory that helps decrease capillary permeability by reducing the number and size of small pores of the capillary walls. The recommendation is 10 to 20 mg taken orally three times a day. It is also available in topical application.

- *Bladder wrack (Fucus vesiculosus)* is a seaweed that has been used historically in cosmetics for its soothing, softening, and toning effects. Topical applications typically contain 0.25 to 75 percent.

- *Cola vera extract* is 14 percent caffeine and has been used topically to help break down fat. Topical applications typically contain 0.5 to 1.5 percent.

Essential Oils: Topical Application

Cellulite Corrector (anticellulite bath)
Blend 1: 8 drops thyme, 4 drops lemon
Blend 2: 8 drops sage, 4 drops patchouli
Blend 3: 6 drops rosemary, 6 drops juniper
Blend 4: 6 drops oregano, 6 drops lemon

Anticellulite Massage Oil Formula
Formula 1: Mix 14 drops juniper with 10 drops lemon and 6 drops oregano.
Formula 2: Mix 8 drops fennel with 10 drops lemon and 12 drops grapefruit.
Formula 3: Mix 10 drops basil with 8 drops thyme and 12 drops grapefruit (use 2 tablespoons almond oil with 5 drops jojoba as a base).
Formula 4: Mix 5 drops juniper with 1 fl. oz, or 25 ml, grapeseed oil (speeds up elimination of waste). Do not use juniper oil if you are pregnant.

JUICE RECOMMENDATIONS

Watermelon, cantaloupe (with seeds), cucumber, parsley, lemon, kiwifruit, and asparagus juices: Natural diuretics

Wheatgrass juice: A powerful body cleanser

Nettles/carrot juice: Excellent for facilitating weight loss, especially on the hips and thighs

The following recipes are suggestions for juice combinations using the fruits and vegetables highest in the nutrients recommended for cellulite.

1. Sources of vitamin C: The Morning Energizer (page 16), Morning Express (page 20), and Beautiful Bone Solution (page 25)

2. Sources of bioflavonoids: Orange Velvet (page 23), Santa Fe Salsa Cocktail (page 19), and Apple Spice (page 36)

3. Helps cleanse the liver: Liver Life Cocktail (page 33) and Popeye's Power (page 21)

4. Good for the thyroid (low thyroid has been connected with cellulite): Radish Care (page 32) and Spicy Tomato on Ice (page 19)

5. Good diuretics: Afternoon Refresher (page 18), Strawberry-Cantaloupe Cocktail (page 38), and Watermelon Refresher (page 40)

HEALTHY HAIR
AND NAILS

HAIR DEVELOPS FROM EPITHELIAL CELLS in the hair follicle, where it receives nourishment from blood vessels in the dermis at the base of the follicle. The bulb region of the follicle contains cells that are important for the regenerative growth of the hair. As older cells grow away from the nutrient supply, they become keratinized and die. These dead epidermal cells become the hair shaft, which grows at a rate of about one-half inch per month. Similarly, the nail plate is produced by specialized epithelial cells that undergo keratinization. A network of capillaries beneath the nail plate are responsible for the nail's pink color. The actively growing portion of the nail (matrix) is thicker and appears white.

Lack of proper nutrition and environmental factors can adversely affect the health of hair and nails, and nutritional deficiencies often show up first in the hair and nails. Not only does good nutrition provide aesthetic benefits to the hair and nails, but by paying attention to these visible signs of nutrient deficiencies, imbalances can be corrected before tissue damage occurs and diseases develop.

DIETARY RECOMMENDATIONS

Protein is important for hair and nail growth and quality. Because hair and nails are made of protein, it is important to eat adequate amounts; too little protein can cause the hair and nails to break off and hair to fall out. However, too much protein and fat can also cause the hair to fall out. Oriental medicine teaches that too much meat will cause hair loss. The best diet is low-fat and high-fiber, with adequate amounts of lean protein. See the Basic Guidelines for the Vibrant Health Diet, page 174. Sulfur-containing amino acids,

L-cysteine and L-methionine, help keratin synthesis, aiding in the growth of hair and nails. Eggs, legumes, and cabbage are the highest sources of sulfur-rich amino acids.

Inadequate intake of protein, vitamin C, and folic acid can lead to hangnails and frayed and split ends of nails. Nails that chip, peel, crack, or break easily indicate a protein and/or hydrochloric acid (HCl) insufficiency. Lack of hydrochloric acid leads to splitting nails. (You can find HCl betaine supplements at most health food stores. HCl should be taken in the middle of a meal.)

NUTRIENT RECOMMENDATIONS

- *Biotin* deficiency can contribute to alopecia (loss of hair). Biotin is not available in appreciable amounts in foods that can be juiced. Best food sources: brewer's yeast, soy products, brown rice, eggs, nuts (especially peanuts, walnuts, and pecans), barley, oatmeal, and sardines.

- *B-complex vitamin* deficiency can cause fragile nails. The B vitamins are responsible for preventing hair loss and graying hair. In general, the best juice source of most B vitamins is green leafy vegetables. Best food sources: whole, unrefined grains such as rye, oats, wheat, buckwheat, and rice, meats, poultry, fish, eggs, nuts, and beans.

- *Vitamin A* (a derivative of retinoic acid) is important for the health of the root and bulb of the hair follicles. In studies, vitamin A was shown to increase hair growth. Dry, brittle nails can also result from a deficiency of vitamin A and calcium. Beta carotene and other carotenoids are converted to vitamin A in the body. Best juice sources of carotenes: carrots, kale, sweet potatoes, parsley, spinach, chard, beet greens, squash, watercress, mangos, sweet peppers, cantaloupes, and apricots.

- *Vitamin D* is involved in the growth and maintenance of hair. Studies point to the presence of vitamin D receptor cells on the hair, noting that they may relate to regulation of hair growth. The body makes vitamin D from sunlight. On a personal note, my hair started growing twice as fast when I moved to sunny Santa Fe, New Mexico, in 1996. My beautician said she had noticed that hair grew faster in this area than in her native Texas. Since we moved to the even sunnier mountains of Colorado, my hair is growing faster than ever. Vitamin D is not available in appreciable amounts in foods that can be juiced—with one exception, sunflower sprouts. Best food sources: sardines, salmon, tuna, shrimp, sunflower seeds, eggs, fortified milk, mushrooms, and natural cheeses.

- *Copper* deficiency may result in white, silver, or gray hair and impaired hair growth. Melanin, the pigment responsible for hair color, is formed in the presence of tyrosinase, an enzyme that utilizes copper as a cofactor. Copper deficiency may also lead to altered pigmentation in the skin. The richest food sources are oysters and lecithin. Best juice sources: carrots, garlic, ginger root, turnips, papayas, and apples.

- *Iron* deficiency in women may lead to heterochromic discoloration of the hair shaft—alternating segments of dark brown and white or silver bands. Low iron tissue stores, even when serum iron levels are normal, can play a role in hair loss. Moderate iron deficiency also can result in fragile fingernails; they can become ridged, lamellated, brittle, or thin and flat, with a spoonlike convexity. Decreased iron absorption can be caused by a lack of hydrochloric acid secretion in the stomach, necessitating supplementation. Best juice sources: parsley, beet greens, chard, dandelion greens, broccoli, cauliflower, strawberries, asparagus, blackberries, cabbage, beets, and carrots.

- *Silicon* deficiency can cause dull, brittle hair and cracked fingernails. This mineral is helpful for keeping your hair from turning prematurely gray. Best juice sources: lettuce, strawberries, mustard greens, parsnips, dandelion greens, cabbage, cucumbers, and alfalfa.

- *Zinc* deficiency can cause white spots on the fingernail bed. Best juice sources: ginger root, parsley, garlic, carrots, grapes, spinach, cabbage, cucumbers, and tangerines.

OTHER RECOMMENDATIONS

Arame is a sea vegetable that is rich in iodine and calcium. It is used traditionally to promote the growth of glossy hair and prevent hair loss.

JUICE RECOMMENDATIONS

Apricot/bell pepper/lettuce/parsley and *carrot juices* are great for promoting shiny hair.

Carrot/lettuce/alfalfa juice and *cabbage/spinach/carrot juice* are used to promote hair growth and to restore hair color.

Carrot/lettuce/spinach juice provides nutrients that are beneficial to the hair root.

Hijiki (seaweed), nettles, and wheatgrass juice are rich in iron and have been used traditionally in the treatment of gray hair. Also, nettles and wheatgrass juice are recommended for prevention of hair loss.

Parsnip/carrot juice adds luster to hair and nails; drink one cup daily.

The following recipes are suggestions for juice combinations using the fruits and vegetables highest in the nutrients recommended for healthy hair and nails.

1. Sources of B vitamins: Sweet Calcium Cocktail (page 24) and Sweet Dreams Nightcap (page 29)

2. Sources of provitamin A (carotenes): The Morning Energizer (page 16) and Beautiful Bone Solution (page 25)

3. Sources of copper: The Ginger Hopper (page 17) and The Immune Builder (page 31)

4. Sources of iron: Popeye's Power (page 21) and The Champ smoothie (page 56)

5. Sources of silicon: Beautiful Skin, Hair, and Nails Cocktail (page 24) and Refreshing Complexion Cocktail (page 25)

6. Sources of zinc: Triple C (page 20) and Grape Expectations (page 40)

Hair-Grow Scalp Massage

Ginger root juice improves circulation and helps to strengthen hair follicles. It's a scalp rejuvenator.

Directions: Juice a 2-inch piece of ginger root and rub the fresh juice into the scalp; leave on for 10 to 15 minutes and rinse with lukewarm water, then shampoo.

Chlorine Cure-All

The combination of lemon and water removes chlorine from the hair and leaves it shiny and clean.

Directions: Mix 1 teaspoon fresh lemon juice in 1 quart water and massage into hair and scalp. Rinse with plain water.

HEALTHY SKIN

HEALTHY, GLOWING SKIN CANNOT BE purchased in a bottle. The best makeup in the world, even applied by a talented makeup artist, can't transform unhealthy-looking skin into a flawless, glowing complexion. Transformation can take place only from the inside out.

Our skin provides protection against environmental damage, such as ultraviolet radiation, and aids in the elimination of toxins from the body. The outer layer of skin (epidermis) receives nourishment from the dermal cells. As epidermal cells divide, they are pushed farther away from the dermis to the surface of the skin. The membranes of the older cells fasten together and undergo *keratinization*—the hardening process in which waterproof proteins develop. The outermost layer of the epidermis is composed of tightly packed dead cells. The skin is continually undergoing a renewal process as these dead cells are sloughed off and new epidermal cells take their place. Because epidermal cells are constantly in a renewal process, there is always hope for a renewed complexion.

Nutrition plays an important role in the maintenance and creation of attractive skin. Your complexion provides an outward picture of your nutritional status and overall health. For many people, subtle nutritional imbalances can manifest themselves quickly in less-than-perfect skin. Healthy eating habits enhance the growth of healthy skin cells, so getting optimal nutrition can transform your skin.

DIETARY AND LIFESTYLE RECOMMENDATIONS

1. *Eat raw fruits and vegetables.* They have enormous potential for improving the skin's appearance. They are one of the reasons that exclusive and expensive health spas worldwide stay in business. Two weeks on a raw-food diet can make a person look 10 years younger—flesh is firmer, lines are softer, and skin, eyes, and hair glow with health. Two years on a high raw-food diet can completely transform the texture, firmness, and contour of the skin. "Living foods" vibrate with a special energy that affects your body internally and externally. To build long-lasting good looks, start with high quantities of fresh raw fruits and vegetables. See Basic Guidelines for the Vibrant Health Diet, page 174.

2. *Juice for great looks!* When freshly made juices are included as part of a high-raw-food diet, they offer remarkable benefits for the skin and over-all appearance. They are loaded with vitamins, minerals, enzymes, phyto-nutrients, and undoubtedly substances not yet discovered, which contribute to healthy, glowing skin. Nutritional deficiencies are common among women. Vitamin/mineral supplements will help, but on their own will not always offer the outstanding benefits most people want. When they are combined with freshly made fruit and vegetable juices, they are far more effective. *All* nutrients are necessary if you are going to look and feel your best, because nutrients are synergistic—each complements the work of another. The average Western diet does not offer enough of these nutrients in the right balance to build long-lasting good looks. But juices are packed with nutrients and are a great supplement to a healthy diet. Consider fresh juices as beautifying dynamos in a glass! See "Drink fresh juice" in Basic Guidelines for the Vibrant Health Diet, page 174.

3. *Try a beauty fast.* Fasting on fresh juices from one to three days is probably the single most effective step you can take to change your appearance. No one has been able to explain why drinking only fresh juices for several days works such a miracle, but "miracle" is the right word. Visible benefits are terrific, including a lessening in the number and depth of facial lines, an improvement in the skin's texture, firmness, and contour, and a vibrant, healthy glow to the skin, eyes, and hair.

Theories as to why fresh juices transform one's appearance echo theories about aging and how to slow that process. At the cellular level, aging is brought about by free-radical damage to cells and an accumulation of wastes and toxins. Wastes build up because of stress and poor nutrition, which impair cellular metabolism and gradually poison and age the body. Drinking only freshly made vegetable and fruit juices for several days is believed to counteract waste buildup by flushing away internal "sludge." When you embark on an internal "spring cleaning" you give your digestive tract a rest and enable immune cells to destroy dead, diseased, or damaged cells. At the same time, the rich concentration of nutrients helps renew your cells.

Every year my husband and I go to the Optimum Health Institute (OHI) of San Diego for a complete internal makeover. We spend a week eating only raw foods, mainly sprouts, with a three-day juice fast in the middle of the week and lots of wheatgrass juice. Everyone jokes about the "OHI glow," but "joke" it is not. In addition to the healthy glow, John and I always leave the institute looking younger and much more vibrant. We might be subjective about how we look, but everyone who knows us comments about the changes when we return home. For more information, see Juice Fasting, page 160.

4. *Care for your skin.*   Cleansing the skin by daily exfoliation and deep-cleansing facial masks keeps the pores clean from debris. Dead cells can accumulate in the skin's pores and cause them to increase in size. Removing makeup properly and using a good skin cleanser can help keep pores from enlarging. Ground sunflower seeds mixed with a small amount of water and rubbed over the skin offers good exfoliation, as does papaya and pineapple pulp. (See Juice and Fruit Pulp Facials, page 94.) Light massage can be beneficial to the skin by increasing circulation and blood and nutrient supply to the dermis. Saunas, exercise, and cold-water splashes make skin glow by removing toxins and improving circulation and suppleness.

NUTRIENT RECOMMENDATIONS

- *Vitamin A and provitamin A (carotenes)* protect the skin against basal cell carcinoma, the most common type of skin cancer. In addition, carotenes give your skin healthy color. Carotenes can be converted by the body to vitamin A as needed. Vitamin A aids in cell growth and is beneficial for treating blemishes and helping to regulate oil balance in the skin. This vitamin also helps combat dry skin by stimulating the renewal of skin cells. Dry skin results from disruptions of the top layer of the epidermis, creating microscopic leaks for moisture to escape. Studies indicate that vitamin A applied to the skin improves elasticity and thickness. Best juice sources: carrots, collard and turnip greens, kale, parsley, spinach, chard, beet greens, watercress, mangos, bell peppers, cantaloupes, apricots, broccoli, and nectarines.

- *Vitamin C* helps improve the skin's suppleness. Vitamin C is a necessary cofactor for the production of collagen, which maintains the elasticity of the skin and gives it firmness and contour. Vitamin C, along with vitamin E, carotenes, and selenium (antioxidants), helps prevent wrinkles by scavenging free radicals that damage cells. Damaged cells contribute to cross-linking of proteins (collagen and elastin) to other molecules. As collagen hardens and elastic tissue diminishes, skin becomes less flexible and more wrinkled and leathery. Research has shown that exposure to ultraviolet radiation depletes the skin of vitamin C, reducing its ability to protect the skin from free-radical destruction caused by sunlight. Best juice sources: kale, parsley, bell peppers, broccoli, Brussels sprouts, watercress, cauliflower, cabbage, strawberries, papayas, spinach, citrus fruits, turnips, mangos, asparagus, and cantaloupes.

- *Bioflavonoids* work synergistically with vitamin C to maximize its potential. Best juice sources: grapes, prunes, citrus fruits, cherries, plums, parsley, cabbage, apricots, bell peppers, papayas, cantaloupes, tomatoes, broccoli, and blackberries.

- *Vitamin E* helps protect against skin cancer, speeds wound healing, and alleviates dry skin. Used topically, vitamin E adds a double helping to improve dryness. Best juice sources: spinach, asparagus, carrots, and tomatoes.

- *Calcium* is important to maintain facial/cranial bone structure. Cranial bone loss can result in sagging skin and wrinkles. Best juice sources: collard and turnip greens, parsley, dandelion greens, watercress, beet greens, broccoli, spinach, romaine lettuce, and green beans.

- *Zinc* is needed to maintain healthy collagen and for production of new collagen. Zinc is essential to help repair tissue and heal scars. It is also useful in the correction of acne. Zinc deficiency can delay wound healing. Best juice sources: ginger, garlic, turnips, parsley, carrots, grapes, spinach, and cabbage.

- *Essential fatty acids* (EFAs) nourish the skin, causing it to look smoother, feel softer, appear more radiant, and remain wrinkle-free longer. Skin nourished with essential fatty acids is infected less easily. EFAs are one of the keys to having skin that is silky to touch and beautiful to photograph. Vegetable juices contain small amounts of EFAs. For more information, see "Fats and Oils" in Diet Guidelines, page 179.

- *Imedeen,* from Scandinavian Naturals, is a protein and glycosamino-glycan concentrate from fish that is recommended by Dr. Julian Whitaker. It can significantly improve the skin's health and help it look younger. Recommended dose is 350 to 500 mg daily. I also recommend *Reguvacare,* a supplement that nourishes the skin and corrects dryness. (It can be ordered from QVC: 800-367-9444.)

JUICE RECOMMENDATIONS

Cabbage juice is used by many cultures to beautify the skin. (Try Triple C, page 20.)

Cucumber and apricot juices are good sources of silicon and are recommended to improve the health and appearance of the skin. The pH of the cucumber is close to that of the skin, and may help prevent wrinkles. Try Afternoon Refresher (page 18).

Bell peppers are good sources of vitamin C and silicon. The juice has been used traditionally to beautify skin, hair, and nails. Try Beautiful Skin, Hair, and Nails Cocktail (page 24).

Dark green lettuce juice mixed with carrot is beneficial in maintaining healthy skin. Try Sweet Dreams Nightcap, page 29.

Parsnip/carrot juice adds luster and softness to skin. Drink 6 to 8 ounces a day with a meal. Try Beautiful Skin, Hair, and Nails Cocktail, page 24.

Green juices, especially wheatgrass juice, are rich in chlorophyll, a blood purifier, which helps prevent skin eruptions. Try Wheatgrass Light, page 21.

The following recipes are suggestions for juice combinations using the fruits and vegetables highest in the nutrients recommended for healthy skin.

1. Sources of carotenes (provitamin A): The Morning Energizer (page 16), The Ginger Hopper (page 17), and Beautiful Bone Solution (page 25)

2. Sources of vitamin C and bioflavonoids: Morning Express (page 20), Popeye's Power (page 21), Orange Velvet (page 23), and Morning Sunrise (page 39)

3. Sources of vitamin E: The Colon Cleanser (page 26), Spring Tonic (page 33), and Spicy Tomato on Ice (page 19)

4. Sources of calcium: Liver Life Cocktail (page 33), Beautiful Bone Solution (page 25), and Parsley Pep (page 26)

5. Sources of zinc: Orient Express (page 18), Ginger Twist (page 17), and Grape Expectations (page 40)

6. Sources of silicon: Refreshing Complexion Cocktail (page 25), Afternoon Refresher (page 18), and Santa Fe Salsa Cocktail (page 19)

The following great-looks cocktails can help improve the condition of the skin. It is recommended that you drink them for three to four weeks.

For the first 12 days drink the following cocktail once a day:

Great Looks Cocktail 1

1 tablespoon artichoke juice (leaves can be juiced)
1 tablespoon stinging nettle juice
1 tablespoon organic dandelion leaf juice
Juice from ½ lemon, peeled if not organic
6 to 8 ounces pineapple or carrot juice

Stir the juice to combine; serve chilled or at room temperature, as desired.

After the twelfth day, drink the following cocktail twice a day for two weeks:

Great Looks Cocktail 2

1 tablespoon stinging nettles juice
1 tablespoon watercress juice
1 tablespoon celery juice
6 to 8 ounces pineapple or carrot juice
1 tablespoon unrefined, organic flaxseed oil (if you don't like the taste
  of this oil, try taking it separately, then "chasing" it with the juice)

Stir the juice to combine; serve chilled or at room temperature, as desired.

JUICE AND FRUIT PULP FACIALS

- *Comfrey juice* is good for dry skin. Juice a handful of comfrey leaves and spread the juice over the face. Leave it on for 10 minutes and rinse with warm water. Follow with a cold-water splash and pat dry.

- *Spinach juice* helps diminish wrinkles. Rub fresh spinach juice in a circular motion around the corners of the eyes, mouth, chin, and across the forehead five times in the morning and five times at night. Rinse your face with cold water and pat dry. This will help to tighten the skin and diminish wrinkles.

- *Freckle Freeze* helps to fade freckles. Blend the juice of 1 lemon with enough granulated sugar to make a paste. Apply to freckled areas; leave it on for 15 minutes and rinse with cool water.

- *Papaya Peeler* is also good to help get rid of freckles. Papaya contains papain, a digestive enzyme that helps break down dead skin cells so they can be washed off. Spread papaya pulp over the face and leave it on for 15 to 25 minutes. Rinse with cool water and pat dry.

- *Pineapple Exfoliator* will help your skin look younger. Pineapple contains the digestive enzyme bromelain. Bromelain is so powerful that pineapple processors must wear industrial-strength rubber gloves when working with the fruit or the enzymes would make their hands raw in a day. This enzyme helps the skin look younger, softer, and less wrinkled. Spread pineapple pulp over your face and leave it on for about 10 minutes. Rinse with cool water and pat dry.

- *After-Tan Moisturizer* will help rehydrate skin cells naturally after a drying day in the sun. Blend the pulp of 2 peaches (drink the juice) with 1 teaspoon of olive oil and make a paste. Leave it on the face 15 minutes. Wash off with cool water.

III

JUICING FOR HIGH-LEVEL WELLNESS

There is a saying that many people spend their health trying to get wealth, only to spend all their wealth to get health. Ralph Waldo Emerson said, "The first wealth is health." If we take time to care for our bodies, we can enjoy that "first wealth."

Wellness is not just the absence of disease, but a state of complete physical, mental, emotional, and social well-being. To me, optimum health means the ability to wake up refreshed each morning, to experience a full day of events without fatigue, to have the energy to accomplish goals, to feel happy and capable of handling challenges, and to be able to meet the demands of life without *dis-ease*.

If you have read my story in the Introduction, you know that health was something I did not have in my childhood and as a young adult in my twenties. Juicing and making other dietary changes gave my body what it needed to heal, cleanse, and be restored.

What does high-level wellness mean to you? Perhaps good health is not something you enjoy today, but something you want to gain. Or maybe you are healthy and you want to preserve what you have, while making some minor improvements.

Fresh juice is an important component to getting or keeping your body in top shape. Juicing and eating smart, along with exercise and a positive outlook, can help you enjoy high-level wellness for many years. Hopefully, for a lifetime.

HIGH-LEVEL ENERGY

IT HAS BEEN CALLED "THE plague of modern civilization"—that lackluster, tired feeling when almost everything is too much effort. Fatigue, characterized by irritability, lethargy, and often malaise, is a common complaint in Western society, yet nearly 80 percent of those who visit their doctors complaining of being chronically tired remain undiagnosed.

Many people are trying to juggle too much responsibility—work, family, school, play, kids' sports, social engagements. You may find that all your responsibilities are making it increasingly difficult to get out of bed in the morning. By midmorning or midafternoon you may feel so tired that you keep reaching for strong cups of coffee and sugary snacks just to keep going. Time and energy for exercise may be nonexistent. Making it through a busy day can be a challenge.

If you lack the energy you want, there is hope. You don't have to be chronically tired. I know. In my twenties I was so fatigued that I could barely walk down the hall in the morning. Even after 12 hours of sleep, I rarely felt rested. Finally, I became so exhausted I couldn't work. Today, I have a schedule of writing, traveling, TV appearances, and speaking engagements that a lot of people in their twenties couldn't keep up with. I encourage you to read my story in the Introduction (page 1), the stories in Carrot Juice for the Soul (page 185), and especially Robyn's story, "A Bank Account for the Future." I think you will be inspired and challenged to change your diet and start juicing for an energetic life.

DIETARY RECOMMENDATIONS

Though for some individuals fatigue may be due to underlying health problems, for most people it is the result of attempting to do too much while at the same time not consuming the right fuel to keep up with energy expenditures. Nutritional deficiencies become more imbalanced with increased activity, because the body needs additional fuel. Also, excessive activity will result in the accumulation of metabolic waste products, and nutrients are needed to detoxify wastes.

Diet plays a central role in providing energy fuel. Making the time to eat smart will increase your energy level, improve your overall mood, help you think more clearly, and give you a greater sense of well-being. If you follow the suggestions here, you should start experiencing a new level of energy in two to three weeks.

1. *Eat a high-fiber, low-fat diet and an abundance of "live" food.*   If you want to feel really alive, eat foods that offer *life.* Raw foods contain a special form of energy derived directly from the sun during photosynthesis. Cooking diminishes that form of energy and destroys vitamins and enzymes. For more information and a suggested menu, see The Vibrant Health Diet, page 174.

2. *Juice your way to high-level energy.*   Fresh juices have demonstrated remarkable qualities for energizing and rejuvenating the body. As you make them part of a largely raw-food diet, you will create a higher level of energy. It is not just the vitamins, minerals, enzymes, phytonutrients, natural hormones, natural antibiotics, and substances yet to be discovered, but also the life force found in the juice that gives you such a power boost. When you drink fresh juice, you are drinking energy converted from the sun. As you continue to juice faithfully—making two or three glasses of juice a part of every day—and eat healthfully, you will most assuredly wake up early one morning, just as I did, without an alarm ringing in your ear, and say to yourself, "This is what it means to feel really *alive!*" I recommend that you do whatever it takes to make fresh juice a part of your lifestyle.

3. *Energy fast!*   Fasting on fresh juices for several days is without a doubt the single most important step you can take to energize your body. It is internal spring cleaning! And it is more important than a tune-up for your car, but I bet you wouldn't put that off too long. A typical Western diet leads to a decline in the interchange of chemicals and energy between the bloodstream and the cells. In a state of good health, cells and capillaries are able to attract what they need and discard what is harmful or unnecessary. But with a fast-food/packaged-food lifestyle, wastes build up in the body, and this selective capacity is diminished. A sticky "marsh" accumulates in the interstitial spaces, and the waste buildup promotes sluggishness and fatigue. A juice fast breaks through this vicious cycle by cleaning out the sludge. It helps the body return to the proper transportation of nutrients and elimination of wastes. During a juice fast, you may feel more tired as the cleansing process goes to work, but after it is over, you will experience a greater sense of vitality and energy.

4. *Avoid refined sugar, caffeine, nicotine, and alcohol.* To achieve a high-energy lifestyle, these substances need to be eliminated. They often provide quick emotional and physical bursts of energy, yet just as quickly leave you feeling burned out. Often, sweets, caffeine, nicotine, and alcohol replace nutritious snacks or meals in a busy person's diet. The I have-no-time-to-eat philosophy deprives the body of essential nutrients and energy sources. These habitual eating patterns leave you exhausted—caught in a destructive cycle of highs and lows.

NUTRIENT RECOMMENDATIONS

- *B-complex vitamins* are important in giving energy by working with enzymes to convert carbohydrates to glucose—the body's source of fuel. In times of stress, they assist the nervous system in functioning optimally. Pantothenic acid, in particular, is important for healthy adrenal gland functioning. When the adrenal glands become exhausted, we feel tired and stressed out; over time, if this vitamin remains deficient, there can be adrenal gland atrophy resulting in extreme fatigue and reduced resistance to allergies and infections. Generally, green leafy vegetables are the best juice sources for most of the B vitamins; pantothenic acid can be found in broccoli, cauliflower, and kale. The best food sources of B vitamins are whole, unrefined grains such as wheat, rice, oats, and rye and meats, poultry, fish, eggs, nuts, and beans.

- *Potassium* is commonly called an *electrolyte* because it carries a small positive electrical charge. Potassium plays a key role in energy metabolism in our bodies. Low levels of potassium are associated with chronic fatigue and exhaustion. This is a mineral that can quickly become deficient in individuals with a high-stress lifestyle who are dependent on quick, pre-prepared foods. Raw fruits and vegetables and fresh juices are loaded with potassium. Best juice sources: parsley, garlic, spinach, broccoli, carrots, celery, radishes, cauliflower, watercress, asparagus, red cabbage, lettuce, cantaloupes, tomatoes, beets, and peaches.

- *Selenium* is a mineral that can help relieve fatigue and energize your body. It is found in the soil in varying degrees; therefore, eating a varied diet of fresh whole foods is the best measure to ensure adequate intake. Studies show that the greater the intake of selenium, the higher the rating of overall mood; the lower the levels of selenium, the more people reported anxiety, depression, and tiredness. Best juice sources: chard, turnips, garlic, oranges, grapes, carrots, and cabbage.

HERBAL RECOMMENDATIONS

Panax ginseng (Korean ginseng) is a common adaptogen (adapts to the body's needs), used widely for improving both physical and mental performance. It is useful for exhaustion and weakness. It has been shown to help individuals deal with very stressful situations and to help increase mental alertness and work output.

Siberian ginseng is used specifically for debility, exhaustion, and depression. It has the ability to increase stamina under all types of stress.

JUICE RECOMMENDATIONS

Specific juices for energy: Wheatgrass is a cereal grass grown from wheat berries. The juice has an abundance of nutrients that are quite helpful in energizing the body. It is recommended that you drink wheatgrass juice straight to achieve maximum benefit; however, many people don't like the taste. If your taste buds need some help, see Wheatgrass Light (page 21).

The following recipes are suggestions for juice combinations using the fruits and vegetables highest in nutrients recommended for energy.

1. Sources of potassium: Popeye's Power (page 21), The Immune Builder (page 31), and Parsley Pep (page 26)

2. Sources of selenium: Morning Express (page 20), Grape Expectations (page 40), and Rise 'n' Shake smoothie (page 55)

LONGEVITY

Do you want to live a long, healthy life? Statistics indicate that people in many European and Asian countries live much longer than Americans. It is believed that our standard American diet (SAD) and toxic environment contribute to the acceleration of aging in this country. Free radicals, which are in part a product of poor diet and a toxic environment, damage cells and greatly contribute to the aging process. Free radicals are highly reactive molecules that lack an electron and attack cells to steal an electron to make them stable, thereby damaging cells in the process. Free-radical damage is implicated in diseases of aging such as atherosclerosis, Alzheimer's and Parkinson's disease, cataracts, and cancer. Preventing free-radical damage through the right dietary choices is one place where we have a great deal of control over how quickly we age.

Surveys show that most baby boomers determine old age to begin at age 79. That is eight years past the average age of life expectancy for men, 71, and one year past that for women. Extending life starts with preventing the causes of premature death such as cardiovascular disease and cancer, while strengthening the systems and organs of the body.

If you want to experience a long and healthy life, start by keeping your body in good health. Since our bodies function on substances found in nature, it makes perfect sense that substances which repair and rejuvenate the body must also be acquired from nature. Most people who have lived over one hundred years, such as Dr. Norman Walker, a pioneer of juicing, have lived a lifestyle based on a diet of unprocessed plant foods that includes plenty of fruits and vegetables.

DIETARY RECOMMENDATIONS

1. *Eat more raw fruits and vegetables and drink an abundance of freshly made juices.* Raw foods have biochemical, physiological, and energizing effects not available in cooked and processed foods. Nearly all cultures noted for their long lives have lived on a diet rich in these kinds of uncooked foods. Raw fruits, vegetables, juices, sprouts, seeds, and nuts are "alive" with energy from the sun made available to us through photosynthesis. They are also rich in vitamins, minerals, enzymes, and phytonutrients—nature's gift to repair and rejuvenate the body.

2. *Avoid sugar, alcohol, and nicotine.* Research indicates that increased amounts of sugar can fuel the aging process; alcohol acts like sugar in the body. Nicotine is known to accelerate aging by generating free radicals and overusing antioxidants in the detoxifying process, which protect the body from the aging processes.

3. *Juice-fast.* Periodic juice-fasts will do wonders to restore and rejuvenate your body. For more information, see Juice Fasting, page 160.

4. *Eat more sparingly and maintain a healthy weight.* Vladimir Dilman, M.D., an authority on antiaging medicine, observed that an increase in body weight is a normal accompaniment of advanced aging. Research with animals has shown that low-calorie diets that are high in nutrients can extend predicted life spans and retard signs of aging. If you want to lose weight, see Weight Loss, page 131.

5. *Improve digestion.* Sometime between the ages of 35 and 45, indigestion becomes a problem for many people. Aging stomachs make less acid and supplementing with HCl betaine or digestive enzymes such as pepsin can be very beneficial in improving digestion. Without adequate hydrochloric acid to activate pepsin, protein won't digest properly and essential amino acids may become deficient. When these and other nutrients are in low supply, enzyme systems, cells, tissues, and organs can't repair themselves and the aging process is accelerated. If you notice your digestion is becoming less efficient, I suggest HCl betaine and/or digestive enzymes (available at most health food stores).

6. *Cleanse and rejuvenate your liver, colon, and kidneys.* These organs of elimination are important to cleanse in order to lengthen your lifespan. Prior to early signs of disease and aging, the efficiency of these organs has often been compromised. Almost every physical problem, such as a lack of energy, skin problems, or sluggish mental functions, have their beginning in poor-functioning organs of elimination. To live a long and healthy life, these organs must be cleansed and strengthened continually. For more information, see the Cleansing Programs, pages 159–173.

NUTRIENT RECOMMENDATIONS

- *Carotenes:* Beta carotene, lycopene, and other carotenes are among the most potent antioxidants. There is scientific evidence that the more carotenes present in tissues, the longer life span. Best juice sources: tomatoes, dandelion greens, carrots, kale, parsley, spinach, beet greens, watercress, mango, cantaloupe, and apricots.

- *Vitamin C,* an antioxidant, is another effective quencher of free radicals. Best juice sources: kale, parsley, broccoli, Brussels sprouts, watercress, strawberries, papayas, spinach, lemons, and grapefruit.

- *Flavonoids* are plant pigments that are responsible for the bright colors of fruits and vegetables. They protect us from free-radical damage and work with vitamin C, making it more effective in your body. Best juice sources: grapes, citrus fruit, cherries, plums, berries, parsley, cabbage, apricots, papayas, and tomatoes.

- *Vitamin E* is an antioxidant that is especially helpful where oxidative stress is involved. Best juice sources: spinach, asparagus, carrots, and tomatoes.

- *Selenium* is an important antioxidant in the fight against aging. Best juice sources: turnips, garlic, oranges, and grapes.

- *Melatonin* is a hormone secreted by the pineal gland that also has antioxidant activity and has been shown to slow the rate of aging and age-related diseases. This supplement can be found at most health food stores.

JUICE RECOMMENDATIONS

Alfalfa sprouts are body cleansers that also help to increase energy and stamina. Try Pure Green Sprout Drink, page 22 (substitute alfalfa sprouts for buckwheat or clover sprouts).

Wheatgrass juice has been shown in studies to inhibit mutations in DNA. Wheatgrass juice is most effective taken alone, but if you have trouble getting used to the taste, try Wheatgrass Light, page 21.

The following recipes are suggestions for juice combinations using the fruits and vegetables highest in the nutrients recommended for longevity.

1. Sources of carotenes: The Ginger Hopper (page 17) and Ginger Twist (page 17)

2. Sources of vitamin C: Strawberry-Cantaloupe Cocktail (page 38) and Morning Express (page 20)

3. Sources of flavonoids: Antiaging Solution (page 39) and Raspberry Sunrise (page 43)

4. Sources of vitamin E: Tomato Florentine (page 22) and Popeye's Power (page 21)

5. Sources of selenium: Morning Sunrise (page 39) and Grape Expectations (page 40)

SEXUAL VITALITY

WHAT INCREASES SEXUAL DESIRE OR the ability to function sexually? Hormones, for one. It is the production of too little testosterone, which declines by an average of 10 percent per decade, that lessens sexual vitality for many people. Women produce testosterone, too. Also, androgen, a substance that stimulates testosterone, varies considerably from one person to another. And for women, lowered progesterone and estrogen also affect sexual desire. In addition, ill health, poor diet, drugs, and psychological issues can diminish libido, whereas good health and a sexual vitality–enhancing diet can increase and/or sustain a healthy sexual drive.

Many men and women are looking for safe and effective ways to increase their sexual drive. Too many reports on the negative side effects of drugs such as Viagra have frightened people. Sex is not worth dying for. But you can be encouraged; there are safe natural remedies that include nutritional supplements, herbs, and foods that are very beneficial.

DIETARY AND LIFESTYLE RECOMMENDATIONS

Both men and women need to be healthy to enjoy a sustained interest in sex. Diet is an important component for sexual vitality. The following suggestions may be helpful for you.

1. *Eat a high-fiber, low-fat diet.* A high-fat, high-cholesterol diet may lead to sexual problems in men by promoting plaque in the penile arteries. Cholesterol blockages are a major reason for impotence. See Basic Guidelines for the Vibrant Health Diet, page 174.

2. *Increase your consumption of freshly made juices and other raw foods.* It is reported that sexual desire tends to improve when more raw foods are included in the diet. Drink two to three eight-ounce glasses of fresh juice daily (more vegetable than fruit) and eat more salads and fresh raw vegetables and fruit.

3. *Avoid alcohol and tobacco.* Alcohol can cause a person to be less sexually responsive and aroused. Smoking tobacco can inhibit sexual function.

4. *Exercise to improve fitness.* A nine-month study of the effect of aerobic exercise on sexuality was completed with 78 healthy but sedentary men. They exercised 60 minutes, 3.5 times a week with a target goal of 70 to 80 percent of their maximum aerobic capacity. Diary entries revealed significantly greater sexuality enhancement in the exercise group. Among the exercisers, positive enhancement was correlated with the degree of individual improvement in fitness. For more information on juicing and fitness, see Exercise and Sports Endurance, page 123.

NUTRIENT RECOMMENDATIONS

Natural substances can boost testosterone levels for men and women and can help restore testosterone, progesterone, and estrogen balance, thus having a very positive effect on sexual vitality.

- *Vitamin C* has been shown to increase sperm count, sperm motility, and sperm viability in men. It is also recommended for men and women who want to increase sexual function. Best juice sources: bell peppers, kale, parsley, broccoli, watercress, cabbage, strawberries, spinach, citrus fruit, and turnips.

- *Rutin,* a flavonoid, has promise in helping to heighten libido and promote a greater orgasmic intensity. Best juice sources: grapes, citrus fruit, cherries, plums, parsley, cabbage, apricots, bell peppers, papayas, cantaloupe, tomatoes, broccoli, and berries.

- *Zinc* assists in the production of testosterone and sperm. Testicular function can be positively affected by zinc. Since oysters are very rich in zinc, this could account for their reputation as aphrodisiacs. Best juice sources: ginger, turnips, parsley, garlic, carrots, grapes, spinach, and cabbage.

HERBAL RECOMMENDATIONS

Avena sativa is obtained from green oats and has been shown to enhance sexual vitality and performance. Scientific tests found that testosterone levels increased from supplementing *Avena sativa*. One study reported enhanced sexual desire, performance, and sensation for both men and women taking *Avena sativa*.

Chaste tree berries can help increase overall sexual vitality. This herb works by balancing the pituitary gland and increasing sexual energy when it is too low.

Damiana is an herb that is considered to be an aphrodisiac. It has been used by Mexican women as a tea taken one hour before intercourse.

Nettles root has been found to inhibit testosterone loss and to help the body in producing more testosterone.

Potency wood is obtained from a shrub found in Brazil and has long been used as an aphrodisiac. Based on scientific studies, it is believed that this herb enhances both the psychological and physical aspects of sexual function.

Wild yam contains a compound called *diosgenin,* which is essentially a progesterone molecule with a smaller molecular addition. Natural progesterone not only protects against facial hair growth and male pattern–type baldness in women, but also improves vaginal dryness. It may require the addition of small amounts of natural estrogen in the form of estriol, which is plant derived, to improve sexual drive in women.

Yohimbine is obtained from the bark of the African yohimbe tree. There is evidence from research with both human and animal studies that yohimbine may have positive effects on sexual performance, including erectile functions as well as desire and arousal.

JUICE RECOMMENDATIONS

Carrots, apples, and ginger have all been shown to help lower cholesterol; try the Ginger Hopper, page 17.

Wheatgrass juice is said to improve sexual functions and desire. It works best when you drink it straight, but if you have trouble getting used to the taste, try Wheatgrass Light, page 21.

The following recipes are suggestions for juice combinations using the fruits and vegetables highest in the nutrients recommended for sexual vitality.

1. Sources of vitamin C: Morning Express (page 20) and Popeye's Power (page 21)

2. Sources of rutin: Tomato Florentine (page 22) and Grape Expectations (page 40)

3. Sources of zinc: Weight Loss Express (page 28) and Sweet Dreams Nightcap (page 29)

IMMUNE SYSTEM SUPPORT

STRENGTHENING AND MAINTAINING A STRONG immune system is crucial to staying healthy. This fascinating system is your first line of defense against disease. It is made up of organs (thymus, spleen, tonsils, adenoids, and lymph nodes), lymphatic vessels, white blood cells (e.g., lymphocytes, monocytes, neutrophils, basophiles, eosinophils), specialized phagocytic cells (e.g., macrophages, reticular cells, leukocytes), and serum factors.

Environmental toxins (pollution, pesticides, cigarette smoke), free radicals, pathogens (yeasts, fungi, parasites), stress, poor dietary habits, nutrient deficiencies (including subclinical), overconsumption of antibiotics, and poor gastrointestinal function all contribute to flagging immunity. When the immune system goes awry, cancer cells can grow undetected, infections can invade and flourish, and other illnesses can develop, echoing factors that cause the body to age.

Free radicals may be a key to the shriveling of the thymus gland, the major gland of the immune system. They also attack immune cells. (Free radicals are unstable molecules that lack an electron and are constantly attacking other cells to steal an electron, thereby setting up a chain reaction creating large numbers of damaged cells.) Signs of a weakened immune system include a greater susceptibility to colds, viruses, flus, infections, and other illnesses.

To most effectively strengthen your immune system, look at all areas of your lifestyle that need improvement. The body is amazingly adaptable. For years we can eat poor foods and appear healthy. But sooner or later, problems manifest. For me it was sooner.

We are told that to stay healthy we must eat a balanced diet, but "balanced diet" to many people means balancing one processed food with another. Consuming a diet with the necessary amounts of nutrients, drinking plenty of pure, clean water, getting regular exercise, and maintaining a healthy outlook on life, along with avoiding toxic substances (e.g., food additives, dyes, and pesticides), is key to healthy immune functions.

DIETARY RECOMMENDATIONS

1. *Eat a high-fiber, low-fat diet.* For a sample menu and guidelines, see Basic Guidelines for the Vibrant Health Diet, page 174.

2. *Avoid sugar and alcohol.* Studies have shown that consuming simple carbohydrates such as glucose, fructose, sucrose, honey, and orange juice all significantly reduced the ability of neutrophils to engulf and destroy bacteria. (Alcohol is a simple carbohydrate.) Because of the high concentration of fruit sugar in fruit juice, limit your intake to no more than 12 ounces per day. Also, it is best to dilute fruit juice by half with water.

3. *Eat more of your vegetables and fruits raw.* Complex carbohydrates should make up the largest portion of your food choices, and of that group, raw vegetables and fruits should compose from 50 to 75 percent of this category. Raw foods are powerful caretakers of the immune system, offering vitamins, minerals, enzymes, essential oils, natural antibiotics, plant hormones, phytonutrients, and various forms of fiber. These raw foods are "alive" with the energy directly derived from the sun during photosynthesis. When we eat the plants, this special energy is passed to our body and thus our immune cells.

4. *Fresh juice equals pure immune power.* Juices provide most of the benefits for the immune system that raw foods do, but with minimum strain on the digestive system. It is estimated that the nutrients are at work in the bloodstream within minutes after drinking them. Some juices have particular immune-enhancing qualities. Wheatgrass juice has been studied for its ability to inhibit mutations in DNA, garlic has antibiotic properties, and ginger is an anti-inflammatory. Cabbage juice is used for its anti-inflammatory, anti-ulcer, and antibiotic qualities.

5. *Juice fasting is a powerful immune booster.* Periodic juice fasting for from one to three days is terrific for getting rid of toxins and waste. It helps the body eliminate poisons at the cellular level, gives the digestive system a rest, and speeds up the white blood cells' ability to destroy diseased, damaged, and dead cells, along with giving the immune system a power boost. If you are not feeling your best, vegetable juice fasting for 24 to 48 hours can greatly benefit your immune system and get you up to speed quickly. (For more information, see Juice Fasting, page 160.)

NUTRIENT RECOMMENDATIONS

- *Vitamin A and carotenes* play a central role in the development of immune cells. Many carotenes, including beta carotene, are converted to vitamin A in the body. Best juice sources: carrots, kale, parsley, spinach, beet greens, watercress, mangos, bell peppers, cantaloupes, and apricots.

- *Vitamin B complex* is especially important for proper immune functioning. Generally, the B vitamins are found in whole grains (such as wheat, rice, oats, and rye), liver, red meat, poultry, fish, eggs, nuts, and beans. The main juice source is green leafy vegetables.

- *Vitamin C* is an antioxidant that can prevent free-radical injury to immune cells. It has been shown to stimulate the immune system and is beneficial in preventing and treating infections and other diseases. It helps activate neutrophils and increases production of white blood cells. Best juice sources: bell peppers, kale, parsley, broccoli, Brussels sprouts, cauliflower, watercress, cabbage, strawberries, papayas, spinach, citrus fruits, mangos, and cantaloupes.

- *Vitamin E* is found in especially high concentrations in the membranes of the immune cells and is essential for normal immune function. It can help prevent free-radical damage to immune cells, which can weaken their ability to respond to challenges. Vitamin E deficiency impairs several aspects of immune response, including B and T lymphocyte and phagocytic activity. Best juice sources: spinach, asparagus, carrots, and tomatoes.

- *Copper* is required for the normal development of immune cells. A low white cell count and immune cell defects can be the consequence of copper deficiency. The typical Western diet provides less copper than is set by the Estimated Safe and Adequate Daily Intake (ESADI) for all age groups. Best juice sources: carrots, garlic, ginger root, turnips, papayas, and apples.

- *Iron* is necessary for healthy red blood cells; a deficiency is immune-suppressive. Best juice sources: parsley, beet greens, chard, dandelion greens, broccoli, cauliflower, strawberries, asparagus, blackberries, cabbage, beets, and carrots.

- *Selenium* is necessary for healthy immune functioning as part of the enzyme activity of glutathione peroxidase. A deficiency may impair immunity. Best juice sources: chard, turnips, garlic, oranges, radishes, grapes, carrots, and cabbage.

- *Zinc* is a mineral necessary for enhanced white blood cell functions. It has been shown to increase T lymphocyte production. Best juice sources: ginger root, parsley, garlic, carrots, grapes, spinach, cabbage, lettuce, cucumbers, and tangerines.

- *Coenzyme Q10* can be made by the body, but we may need more than the body can make at times of immunological stress. Coenzyme Q10 (CoQ10) has a number of immune-enhancing effects, including increasing phagocytic activity and proliferation of granulocytes. Age-related immune decline may be reversed with CoQ10 supplementation. Best food/juice sources: beef heart, sardines, peanuts, and spinach. (CoQ10 supplements can be found at health food stores.)

- *Glutathione* is an antioxidant important to lymphocyte reproduction and T cell function. It is essential in recycling oxidized vitamins E and C. Best juice sources: asparagus, watermelon, citrus fruits, strawberries, peaches, cauliflower, broccoli, and tomatoes.

HERBAL RECOMMENDATIONS

Astragalus has been shown in studies to restore immune function when the immune system is suppressed. It has also been shown to increase antibody and interferon production and increase T helper cell activity.

Echinacea is immune-enhancing and has antiviral activity. It provides an immune-stimulating boost.

JUICE RECOMMENDATIONS

Wheatgrass juice: Best taken straight, but some people don't like the taste, in which case, try Wheatgrass Light, page 21

Garlic has antiviral properties. See The Immune Builder, page 31

Ginger root is rich in zinc. See The Morning Energizer, page 16
Cabbage juice is a traditional remedy used to build up the immune system.
   See Triple C, page 20

The following recipes are suggestions for juice combinations using the fruits and vegetables highest in the recommended nutrients for the immune system.

1. Sources of glutathione: Just Peachy (page 37), Strawberry-Cantaloupe Cocktail (page 38), and Morning Sunrise (page 39)

2. Sources of iron: Popeye's Power (page 21) and Liver Life Cocktail (page 33)

3. Sources of selenium: Morning Express (page 20), Radish Solution (page 30), and Grape Expectations (page 40)

4. Sources of provitamin A (carotenes): Beautiful Skin, Hair, and Nails Cocktail (page 24) and Mango Mania smoothie (page 57)

5. Sources of vitamin C and bioflavonoids: Beautiful Bone Solution (page 25) and Parsley Pep (page 26)

6. Sources of vitamin E: Spring Tonic (page 33) and The Colon Cleanser (page 26)

7. Sources of zinc: The Ginger Hopper (page 17) and Antiaging Solution (page 39)

PEAK MEMORY
AND MENTAL PERFORMANCE

MEMORY AND COGNITION CAN BE improved as can the ability to focus mentally and utilize one's mental capacities successfully on demand. Symptoms of poor mental performance include impaired learning ability, poor recall of information, and difficulty following conversation or train of thought.

To improve memory, you must have adequate nutrition and amino acid balance, and address, if necessary, allergies, candidiasis, parasites, thyroid disorders, low blood sugar, and poor circulation to the brain.

General decline in mental performance and actual damage to brain cells and shrinkage of the brain is caused most often by free-radical damage. Free radicals are highly reactive molecules that lack an electron; they attack cells to steal an electron to make them stable and damage cells in the process. Damaged cells then become free radicals, and a chain reaction is set in motion. Free-radical attack on proteins in the brain turns them into sludge called *lipofuscin*—a form of brown slime that can coat neurons. As the slime thickens, memory declines. Free-radical damage to the hypothalamus and pituitary glands results in a decline in growth hormone (GH); free-radical attack on the adrenal glands results in a decline in the hormone DHEA— these hormones may be essential to the ability to learn and form memories. Due to a host of modern-world pollutants, processed foods, computers and other sources of low-electromagnetic-field toxicity, and other generators of free radicals, many middle-aged and even younger people are suffering declines in intelligence, ability to learn, memory, and capacity to think clearly.

Peak mental performance is a necessity for many people. Business meetings require that you be in top form. There are reports to go over, facts to memorize, summaries to write. Your job demands an alert, quick mind. You want to stop any mental decline and get your brain in top shape.

Your first step? Scavenge free radicals and prevent attacks on brain cells with an abundance of antioxidant nutrients. And feed your body high-quality "brain food" every day. Whether you want to improve memory performance or enhance creativity, concentration, and alertness, and prevent brain aging—dietary boosters from juicing and nutritional supplements can make a tremendous difference.

DIETARY RECOMMENDATIONS

How we think has a lot to do with how we eat. Eating well has been proven to improve mental performance and cognitive function. For example, a number of studies have confirmed that school breakfast programs have a positive effect on helping disadvantaged children to learn. This leads one to wonder what benefit the typical morning cup of coffee and doughnut could possibly give the brain.

1. *Eat a high-fiber, low-fat diet.* An all-carbohydrate meal can adversely affect memory. For best mental performance, combine complex carbohydrates (vegetables, whole grains, legumes) with 10 to 15 percent protein and 15 to 25 percent essential fatty acids. (Essential fatty acids can help improve mental functions.) For a sample menu and guidelines, see Basic Guidelines for the Vibrant Health Diet, page 174.

2. *Avoid refined sugars and alcohol*—they "turn off" the brain.

3. *Juicing and juice fasting* help the body get rid of brain sludge (lipofuscin) and prevent free-radical attacks on brain cells. Fresh juices are loaded with antioxidants that bind to the "wild bullet" molecules known as free radicals so that they cannot damage your brain. Juice fasting for several days gives the body a chance to do a thorough "spring cleaning" on the brain. Many people say that after a juice fast they feel much more alert and alive and can think more clearly. (For more information, see the section on Juice Fasting, page 160, and other Cleansing Programs, pages 159–173.)

NUTRIENT RECOMMENDATIONS

Some tests have shown that certain nutrients will improve cognitive functions. One study was done with children 6 to 60 months old who were given daily nutritional supplementation for three months. Eight years later they were tested to measure memory function. The children 18 months and younger who had been given the supplements performed better than those who did not receive nutritional supplementation. Research shows that a deficiency of certain nutrients can cause memory and learning problems. Supplying the right nutrients can stop a decline in mental function as well as improve overall mental performance.

The brain draws memories from the storage area to your conscious mind via substances called *neurotransmitters*—electrochemical messengers that stimulate your memory—such as acetylcholine (ACh), epinephrine, and serotonin. You can improve neurotransmitter status with nutrients that support them. Overall brain function can be enhanced by consuming a generous supply of nutrients that empower brain functions and protect the brain from free-radical damage.

- *Choline.* Acetylcholine is *the most important* neurotransmitter for memory and intelligence—your body makes it from choline, one of the B vitamins. Some studies show that choline has improved memory dramatically in healthy young adults. In times of stress, choline has provided an immediate boost in brainpower. There is also evidence that choline can improve mental functioning and thought transmission by strengthening neurons in the brain's memory centers and slowing down age-related loss of dendrites. Choline is found in highest quantities in lecithin. (Lecithin capsules and granules can be purchased at most health food stores.) Best juice sources: green beans, cabbage, spinach, and oranges.

- *Vitamin C* is a potent cognitive-enhancing antioxidant that can boost brainpower. One study has shown vitamin C supplementation, given to those with low levels of this vitamin, increased IQ scores over 3.5 points. Best juice sources: bell peppers, kale, parsley, broccoli, Brussels sprouts, cauliflower, cabbage, strawberries, papayas, spinach, citrus fruits, mangos, and cantaloupes.

- *Boron* is a trace mineral that has yet to be recognized as essential for human beings; however, deficiencies have been noted to affect cognitive performance. A set of three studies found that low intake of boron resulted in significantly poorer performance on tasks involving encoding, short-term memory, and attention. Fruits and vegetables are the best sources of boron; therefore, you have a wide variety of juices from which to choose.

- *Glutathione* is a brain-enhancing substance that increases the flow of blood and oxygen to the brain. It has a protective effect on the brain's cells and boosts mental functions. Best juice sources: asparagus, watermelon, citrus fruits, strawberries, peaches, cauliflower, broccoli, tomatoes, and avocados (avocados don't juice well, but they make a great raw soup base; see Cherie's Quick-Energy Soup, page 62).
- *Other brain boosters.* A number of amino acids such as glutamine, phenylalanine, pyroglutamate, methionine, and threonine have been shown to enhance learning and memory. Other substances such as N-acetyl-L-carnitine and DMG may also be helpful. For more information on brainpower nutrients, see *Mega Brain Power* by Michael Hutchinson (Hyperion, 1994).

HERBAL RECOMMENDATIONS

Ginkgo biloba increases the flow of blood and oxygen to the brain and helps the brain more efficiently utilize blood glucose (glucose is the brain's primary source of fuel and energy). Studies show that ginkgo increases the brain's alpha rhythms—brain wave frequencies associated with absence of stress and calm alertness—while decreasing theta activity (associated with drowsiness and an inability to concentrate).

JUICE RECOMMENDATIONS

The following recipes are suggestions for combinations using the fruits and vegetables highest in the recommended nutrients for brainpower.

1. Sources of choline: Popeye's Power (page 21), The Memory Mender (page 27), and The Champ smoothie—add lecithin for a powerful helping of choline (page 56)

2. Sources of glutathione: Spring Tonic (page 33), Watermelon Refresher (page 40), and Spicy Peaches 'n' Cream smoothie (page 59)

3. Sources of vitamin C: Beautiful Skin, Hair, and Nails Cocktail (page 24), Strawberry-Cantaloupe Cocktail (page 38), and Tropical Sunrise smoothie—add lecithin for an extra boost of choline (page 55)

ENHANCING JOB PERFORMANCE

HOW WELL YOU PERFORM OR don't perform on the job could mean the difference between a promotion, a demotion, or even worse. If you are often sick or you are tired and can't produce the work expected, your job could be in jeopardy. Conversely, if you are full of energy, rarely sick, mentally alert, and you work efficiently, you will be a valued employee.

Nutrition plays an important part in job performance. When you feed your body super food, it has the best chance of functioning at peak levels. It's similar to adding premium fuel to your gas tank. When you do, you know your car will run better than on cheap fuel. The harder you work, the more high-quality food your body needs to function at its top physical level and to increase your stamina and endurance. To increase mental capacity for writing, research, speech preparation, and other cognitive functions, you also need brain food. For more information, see Peak Memory and Mental Performance, page 116.

DIETARY RECOMMENDATIONS

1. *Increase complex carbohydrates,* especially vegetables. Carbohydrates can help improve performance when combined with high-quality lean protein. For more information, see the Vibrant Health Diet, page 174.

2. *Eat more high-performance foods.*   To reach a high level of job performance, make raw fruits, vegetables, juices, sprouts, nuts, and seeds at least 50 percent of your diet. These foods are "alive" with the energy from the sun derived through photosynthesis. Cooking diminishes that energy and also destroys vitamins and enzymes.

Fresh juice in particular can directly improve your performance on the job. The executives I've known who keep a juicer at the office, juice during the day, and encouraged their employees to make fresh juice, claim they and their employees have experienced more energy, stamina, and mental clarity than when they didn't juice. And they also observed better job performance and fewer sick days among their employees. If you experience low energy midmorning or midafternoon, have trouble concentrating at times, or become fatigued before you have finished a project, fresh juice breaks are super pick-me-ups that can make a significant difference in your workday.

3. *Avoid refined sugar, caffeine, nicotine, and alcohol.* These substances rob your energy. They often provide quick emotional and physical bursts of energy, yet just as quickly leave you feeling depleted. They keep you on a physical and emotional cycle of highs and lows. Also, these substances can replace nutritious snacks or meals when you are busy and will deprive you of essential nutrients and energy sources.

NUTRIENT RECOMMENDATIONS

- *B complex vitamins* are important for the healthy functioning of the nervous system. Pantothenic acid, in particular, is very helpful for stress because it supports the adrenal glands. When the adrenal glands become overworked, you feel tired, irritable, and stressed out. The best juice sources, generally, are leafy green vegetables for B vitamins; pantothenic acid can be found in broccoli, cauliflower, and kale.

- *Choline* can help reduce fatigue and improve muscle performance. Best juice sources: green beans, cabbage, spinach, and oranges.

- *Potassium* is involved in energy metabolism. It can quickly become deficient in individuals leading a high-stress lifestyle. Generally, raw fruits and vegetables and fresh juices are the richest sources of potassium. Best juice sources: parsley, garlic, spinach, broccoli, carrot, celery, radish, cauliflower, watercress, asparagus, red cabbage, and lettuce.

- *Selenium* is a mineral that helps improve energy. Studies show that the greater the intake of selenium, the more improvement in overall mood; conversely, the lower the levels of selenium, the more people reported anxiety, depression, and tiredness. Best juice sources: chard, turnips, garlic, oranges, grapes, carrots, and cabbage.

- *Tyrosine,* an amino acid present in many proteins, has an effect on nerve impulse transmission and may improve vigilance and lessen anxiety. Vitamin C and folic acid are essential for the metabolism of tyrosine. Eat high-quality protein for tyrosine and drink juices rich in vitamin C and folic acid. Best juice sources of vitamin C: kale, parsley, broccoli, cauliflower, cabbage, strawberries, papaya, spinach, oranges, mangos, asparagus, and cantaloupe. Best juice sources of folic acid: asparagus, spinach, kale, broccoli, cabbage, blackberries, and oranges.

HERBAL RECOMMENDATIONS

Panax ginseng (Korean ginseng) is used for improving both physical and mental performance and for exhaustion and weakness. It helps increase mental alertness and work output and helps individuals deal with stressful situations.

Siberian ginseng has been shown to increase stamina under stressful conditions.

JUICE RECOMMENDATIONS

The following recipes are suggestions for juice combinations of the fruits and vegetables highest in the recommended nutrients for peak job performance.

1. Sources of choline: Popeye's Power (page 21) and Triple C (page 20)

2. Sources of folic acid: Sweet Calcium Cocktail (page 24) and Spring Tonic (page 33)

3. Sources of pantothenic acid: Magnesium Special (page 22) and The Memory Mender (page 27)

4. Sources of vitamin C: Beautiful Bone Solution (page 25) and Morning Express

5. Sources of potassium: Parsley Pep (page 26) and The Morning Energizer (page 16)

6. Sources of selenium: Apple Spice (page 36) and Snappy Ginger (page 38)

EXERCISE AND SPORTS ENDURANCE

THE HEALTH BENEFITS OF REGULAR exercise cannot be overstated. In response to continual exercise, the body becomes stronger and more efficient and has greater endurance. Regular exercise improves cardiovascular and respiratory functions. Aerobic exercise such as walking or running enhances the transport of nutrients and oxygen into the cells. At the same time it facilitates shuttling carbon dioxide and waste materials from the tissues to be eliminated.

According to the Surgeon General's 1996 report, regular physical exercise reduces the risk of dying from coronary heart disease and of developing type II diabetes, hypertension, and colon cancer. It enhances mental health, improves muscle tone, and strengthens bones and joints. Tension, stress, depression, anxiety, and worry diminish significantly with regular exercise. The reward of exercise, a healthy diet, and a positive attitude is a very high level of energy, happiness, vitality, and passion for life. In light of all the benefits, it is surprising that more than 60 percent of Americans don't exercise regularly and 25 percent don't exercise at all.

To increase energy for exercise and conditioning, see the chapter on High-Level Energy (page 99). In addition, pay attention not only to the fuel reserves in the muscle, but also to the muscle's ability to use that fuel. Vitamins, minerals, and other nutrients are key to that process. The best way to put nutrients into your body is to eat a well-balanced diet with enough calories to meet your expenditures. Even with the best intentions, however, you may fall short—busy schedules, weight-loss programs, or food intolerances can keep you from getting all the nutrition you need. Fresh fruit and vegetable juices can fill in the gaps by providing you with easily absorbed vitamins, minerals, enzymes, and phytonutrients in delicious form.

AEROBIC EXERCISE

Aerobic exercise is defined as any exercise during which the energy needed is supplied by oxygen intake. Whether you walk, jog, take an aerobic dance class, or try step aerobics, you will need to supply your body with the nutrients it needs for get-up-and-go so you can use the oxygen you are inhaling.

Dietary Recommendations

Follow the Basic Guidelines for the Vibrant Health Diet, page 174.

Nutrient Recommendations

All nutrients are important for exercise; however, some vitamins and minerals, such as the antioxidants (vitamins C and E, beta carotene, and selenium), are particularly beneficial as scavengers of free radicals. Free radicals are molecules with an unpaired electron looking to steal an electron from another cell, thereby damaging it. Antioxidants may be particularly helpful in minimizing muscle soreness for the weekend athlete and older individuals who exercise vigorously. Unaccustomed exercise may result in delayed-onset muscle soreness due to microscopic tears in the muscle; antioxidants can help prevent or heal these tears. Antioxidants also help control the free radicals and lipid peroxidation that normally occur following the rise in oxygen consumption with exercise.

The following antioxidants and other nutrients can help to energize your exercise routine.

- *Beta carotene* is a fat-soluble antioxidant that is *the most effective* single oxygen quencher (an oxygen-free radical). Exercise can generate more of these free radicals. Best juice sources: dandelion greens, carrots, kale, parsley, spinach, turnip greens, chard, beet greens, watercress, mangos, red peppers, and cantaloupes.

- *B vitamins* are the metabolic regulators. Some B vitamins directly coordinate energy, and your need for them is proportional to expenditure. Eating a diet high in complex carbohydrates such as vegetables, legumes, whole grains, and fruit, plus lean animal protein for vitamin B_{12}, is your best assurance of getting ample amounts of these vitamins. Juicing dark leafy greens such as kale, spinach, and parsley will offer added B vitamins, such as B_2, which may be needed in higher quantities to meet muscle demands. Vitamin B_1 plays an important role in carbohydrate metabolism. The need for vitamin B_6 is increased with higher dietary protein intake and the high turnover rate of muscle cells. For vitamin B_6, eat more fish, chicken, beans, whole grains, nuts, seeds (especially sunflower), bananas, and avocados, and drink juices made with kale and spinach.

- *Vitamin C* helps protect against exercise-induced damage to muscle tissue. Vitamin C works as a water-soluble antioxidant. Best juice sources: kale, parsley, green peppers, broccoli, Brussels sprouts, watercress, cauliflower, red and green cabbage, strawberries, papayas, spinach, citrus fruits, turnips, mangos, and asparagus.

- *Vitamin E* can improve immune response, which will stimulate faster muscle repair. Vitamin E is an antioxidant that decreases the production of oxygen-free radicals. Studies show that exercise can increase lipid peroxidation—free-radical damage to fats and cholesterol (lipids) within the body; this process accelerates at high altitude. When lipids are damaged, they form toxic by-products known as *lipid peroxides* and *cholesterol epoxides*. Studies show that vitamin E supplementation at 200 mg twice a day inhibits lipid peroxidation. Best juice sources: spinach, asparagus, carrots, and tomatoes.

- *Potassium* deficiency can cause muscle weakness, problems with muscle contraction, and fatigue. Best juice sources: parsley, yams, chard, garlic, spinach, and broccoli.

- *Zinc* is needed for energy metabolism. Theoretically, low zinc levels would result in reduced endurance capacity, and zinc deficiency is related to muscular fatigue. Best juice sources: ginger root, turnips, parsley, potatoes, garlic, and carrots.

Herbal Recommendations

Ginseng has been used for thousands of years in the Orient as a tonic and restorative agent. It has also been used by athletes for its positive effects on performance.

Ginger root has anti-inflammatory properties that could be helpful with muscle soreness.

Juice Recommendations

The following recipes are suggestions for combinations using the fruits and vegetables highest in the recommended nutrients for exercise.

1. Sources of beta carotene and vitamin B_1: The Morning Energizer (page 16), Popeye's Power (page 21), and Beautiful Bone Solution (page 25)

2. Sources of vitamin B_6: Tropical Sunrise (page 55), Rise and Shake (page 55), The Champ (page 56), all smoothies, and Cherie's Quick-Energy Soup (page 62)

3. Sources of vitamin C: Morning Express (page 20), Beautiful Bone Solution (page 25), and Strawberry-Cantaloupe Cocktail (page 38)

4. Sources of vitamin E and potassium: Muscle Power Plus smoothie (page 56), The Colon Cleanser (page 26), and Spring Tonic (page 33)

5. Sources of zinc: The Ginger Hopper (page 17), Ginger Twist (page 17), Waldorf Twist (page 16), The Immune Builder (page 31), and Apple Spice (page 36) (ginger root can help inflammation and soreness)

STRENGTH AND ENDURANCE SPORTS

While moderate exercise is beneficial for the immune system and overall health, exhaustive exercise can lead to an increased production of free radicals and thus to impaired immune function, greater exposure to infections, cancer, and aging. If you are involved in strenuous exercise or endurance sports, pay particular attention to the antioxidants—vitamins C, E, and A, the carotenes, coenzyme Q10, and glutathione. Though these nutrients may not make a noticeable difference in your performance, they can prevent free-radical damage by scavenging those "wild bullet" free radicals that attack cells and cause oxidative damage.

Dietary Recommendations

Follow the basic guidelines in the beginning of this section, which apply to all exercise. In addition, incorporate the following specific points that apply to your needs.

1. *Consume 60 to 65 percent of your calories from complex carbohydrates.* Carbohydrates fuel muscles for exercise, promote muscle growth, and increase the chance that the weight you gain will be more muscle than fat. You should replace the carbohydrates in your muscles within 30 minutes to two hours after exercise. Choose quality carbohydrates such as whole-grain cereals, bananas, vegetable-fruit juice combinations, whole-grain pasta, brown rice, beans, lentils, split peas, and vegetables (and make sure a large percentage of your vegetables and fruits are raw—see the Vibrant Health Diet, page 174).

2. *Increase your protein intake.*   Protein requirements are higher when a person is involved in strength and endurance exercises. Extra protein can aid strength training by helping build muscle and may promote endurance by replacing protein that is oxidized for energy during exercise. Athletes who use strength, power, and speed need to consume between .6 and .8 grams of protein per pound of body weight per day, and endurance athletes need .5 to .6 grams. Multiply your body weight (pounds) by one of these numbers to find out how much protein you should eat. Figure grams of protein as follows: 1 cup of milk or 1 egg contains 8 grams of protein; 1 ounce of beef, chicken, fish, nuts, seeds, or ½ cup dried beans contains 7 grams. There is no evidence that more protein than this will give you additional muscle-building advantage.

Some athletes have switched to more vegetarian diets and have become protein deficient. Strict vegans need to consume more whole grains, beans, lentils, split peas, and soy products. Protein-deficiency signs include hair falling out and growing slowly, or breaking and peeling fingernails. Endurance athletes may actually use more protein than bodybuilders.

3. *Drink your vegetables.*   Carrot juice and other vegetable juices can give you muscle-building advantage. Just ask Gary Liss, bodybuilder and personal trainer. He proudly states that he built his strong body on carrot juice. Read his story "You Are What You Eat" in the section "Carrot Juice for the Soul," page 185, and see the section on juicing and raw foods in Basic Guidelines for the Vibrant Health Diet, page 177.

Nutrient Recommendations

- *Vitamin C* levels have been shown to be reduced by approximately 20 percent in runners following a 21-km race; 600 to 1,000 mg of vitamin C is recommended for about two months prior to an event to lower the risk of postexercise respiratory infection. Be sure to take supplemental C with juices high in vitamin C and bioflavonoids (phy-tonutrients) to supply plenty of "cofactors" that make vitamin C more effective. Best juice sources of vitamin C: kale, parsley, collard and turnip greens, red peppers, broccoli, Brussels sprouts, watercress, cau-liflower, cabbage, strawberries, papayas, spinach, citrus fruits, turnips, mangos, asparagus, and cantaloupes. Best juice sources of bioflavonoids: grapes, citrus fruits, cherries, plums, parsley, grape-fruit, cabbage, apricots, bell peppers, papayas, cantaloupes, tomatoes, and broccoli.

- *Chromium* can help increase body mass. One study of students taking chromium at 200 micrograms (mcg) a day increased lean tissue by 1.6 kg, while that of subjects taking a placebo (0 mcg) increased body mass by only .04 kg during a 40-day weight-lifting study. Best juice sources: potatoes, green bell peppers, apples, parsnips, spinach, and carrots.

- *Magnesium* plays a significant role in protein synthesis. In a double-blind, seven-week, strength-training-program study, about half of the untrained athletes were given magnesium oxide supplements. Both groups gained strength, but there was a significant difference in torque gain with the magnesium group. Best juice sources: beet greens, prunes, chard, collard greens, and parsley.

- *L-carnitine* is an amine that is synthesized from two essential amino acids—lysine and methionine. A study published in 1997 with marathon runners showed that L-carnitine supplements positively influenced aerobic capacity with normal lipid (fat) levels. Carnitine production is enhanced in the body by consuming vitamin C and lysine. Best food sources: meat and dairy products. (It is not available in appreciable amounts in juice sources.)

Juice Recommendations

See the section on exercise for a variety of helpful recipe ideas. In addition, add the following recipes that are suggested for juice combinations highest in the recommended nutrients for strength and endurance sports:

1. Sources of beta carotene, vitamin C, zinc, magnesium, and chromium: Strawberry-Almond Surprise (page 60), Berry Smooth (page 58), Muscle Power Plus (page 57), all smoothies, and The Morning Energizer (page 16)

2. Sources of chromium: The Colon Cleanser (page 26), Beautiful Hair, Skin, and Nails Cocktail (page 24), and Popeye's Power (page 21)

3. Drink Nature's Best Electrolyte Replacer (page 46) instead of commercial drinks that contain refined sugar and preservatives

PRE- AND POST-EVENT TIPS

Carbohydrate loading is a plan to follow the week before a competition. Many sports nutrition specialists say it can give you a competitive edge. Endurance cyclists have demonstrated that loading up on carbohydrates can improve power and speed. Carb loading, as it is called, is effective only for endurance competition lasting 90 minutes or more. The strategy is to rest your muscles before the race, called *tapering,* and to eat lots of complex carbohydrates and minimal fat. The best foods to consume are beans, whole grains, and vegetables plus vegetable juices. You may put on two to four pounds before the event, which means the carb loading worked. It is important to consume plenty of fluids when you load carbohydrates—at least eight 8-ounce glasses of fluid (this can include both water and juice).

On days 6 through 4 before the event, make 60 percent of your food complex carbohydrates. On day three, increase your carbohydrates to 70 percent.

Two Days Before the Event

Train lightly, about 20 minutes, and eat 70 percent complex carbohydrates. Minimize salt and salty food. Avoid caffeine and alcohol. Drink plenty of fluids—water and fresh juices.

One Day Before the Event

Train lightly, about 20 minutes, and eat 80 percent carbohydrates; but decrease foods that are high in fiber and reduce your solid food intake. Drink more fresh vegetable juices. For endurance events, reduce your protein intake—excess protein increases elimination of urine and leads to dehydration. Obtain more calories from fresh juices, especially vegetable juices; minimize fruit juice to prevent a hypoglycemic reaction, and dilute fruit juices with water.

Day of the Event

On the day of the race, you should rest and eat a 70 percent carbohydrate meal. Solid food intake should be light carbohydrates such as cream of brown rice cereal; high-fiber meals require energy to digest and can make you feel full and sluggish. Unless you know you won't react, avoid bananas, celery, grapes, peaches, and shrimp before the event—these foods can cause allergic reactions in some people, and strenuous exercise increases the absorption of allergens. Stop eating 2½ hours prior to the race. Up until one hour before the race, drink at least 16 ounces of water and/or juice diluted with half water. From one hour to 15 minutes before the event, drink no fluids; 15 minutes prior to the race, drink 8 ounces of water.

If the event lasts longer than 60 minutes, you will need to replace electrolytes. Drink ½ cup of Nature's Best Electrolyte Replacer, page 46, every 20 minutes. For all-day races or multiday events, a more concentrated commercial sports drink should be alternated with Nature's Best Electrolyte Replacer. Use a commercial drink altogether if you are in immediate danger of exhaustion—the sweetener is from glucose or sucrose, which is absorbed more quickly than fruit sugars.

Post-event

When your heart rate falls below 100 beats per minute, you can begin taking fluids, calories, and nutrients. Drink potassium-rich juices made with parsley, spinach, carrots, and apples; eat a banana or make a smoothie with a banana. For juice and smoothie recipes, see pages 35–62. Eat complex carbohydrates such as brown rice, vegetables, and beans to replace glycogen, which is broken down into lactic acid during exercise.

WEIGHT LOSS

WHO DOESN'T WANT TO LOSE a few pounds? Most people would like to lose weight at almost any time in their life. Right now, 99 million Americans are overweight, and obesity is considered the second-leading cause of death in the United States. Anyone who is 20 percent over the recommended weight for his or her age, build, and height is considered obese.

Whether you want to lose just a couple of pounds or 20, 50, or more, weight loss takes a commitment. No magic is involved. There is only one way to reach your goal—burn more calories than you take in. To do this, you must eat smart by making your calories count for energy (empty calories are most likely to get stored as fat) and get regular exercise.

DIETARY RECOMMENDATIONS

1. *Eat a low-fat diet.* Studies show that fat leads to weight gain. People who are overweight are less prevalent in places where the traditional diet is low in fat—for example, in China and Japan. Fat is stored more efficiently than carbohydrates or protein; it enters the body in storage form. A study published in 1997 found that those who ate a low-fat, high-carbohydrate meal consumed an average of 680 calories, while those who ate a high-fat meal did not feel full until they had consumed 1,350 calories. There are nine calories in one fat gram versus four calories in one gram of protein or carbohydrate. Make sure your fat intake is 25 percent or less of your total calories, and of that fat, make sure more than half is unsaturated. (For more information, see "Fats and Oils" under the Vibrant Health Diet Guidelines, page 177.)

2. *Increase fiber.* A high-fiber diet increases "bulk" and gives a feeling of fullness, making it less likely you will overeat. Foods high in fiber are relatively low in calories and provide consistent energy production. A high-fiber diet supports good colon function and helps eliminate wastes and toxins released in weight loss. Fiber actually reduces the number of calories the body absorbs. In some clinical studies showing weight loss, supplemental fiber reduced the number of calories absorbed by 30 to 180 calories a day. Fiber taken immediately before a meal can be beneficial in reducing appetite. The best forms of fiber are psyllium husk powder, guar gum, and pectin—all are water-soluble fibers. Mix fiber in fresh juice or water and drink it before a meal or in between meals. (Avoid fiber products that contain sugar or other sweeteners.)

3. *Fresh juice facilitates weight loss.* I have received numerous letters from people who have used the weight-loss suggestions in my first juice book to lose 10, 20, or more pounds. One individual lost 150 pounds by incorporating fresh juice into his weight-loss plan. (Dilute fruit juice with water to lower calories and prevent appetite stimulation from the fruit sugars.)

A great weight-loss/maintenance program, and one I use continually, is a one-day-a-week juice fast. Drink only fresh juices, mainly vegetable juices, all day and eat no solid food. I often make my Quick-Energy Soup (page 62) for lunch or dinner. You will not only lose a pound or two that week, but you'll feel energized and renewed. And if you want a powerful jump start to your weight-loss program, begin with a two- or three-day juice fast. (See the section on Juice Fasting, page 160.) Fresh juice facilitates weight reduction for a variety of reasons:

- *Fresh juice is chock-full of nutrients* that feed your body, and it is already broken down into an easily absorbed form so you will receive its energizing benefits right away. When you don't get the proper nutrients, your body continues to send you hunger signals. Do you ever wander through the kitchen wanting something more to eat, but you don't know what it is? Cravings diminish when you are fed an abundance of absorbable nutrients.

- *Fresh juice is very low in calories* and has virtually no fat. For example, The Ginger Hopper, page 17, has only 196 calories and 0 calories from fat.

- *Many juices are natural diuretics* that help you excrete excess water. Watermelon, cucumber, parsley, asparagus, lemon, kiwifruit, and cantaloupe juice, with seeds, all contain diuretic properties.

- *Juice contains soluble fiber* that can improve the intestinal muscle's ability to push waste through the gastrointestinal tract. Pectins (soluble fiber found in juices) also bind to and eliminate toxins in the gut.

4. *Drink at least 64 ounces of water daily.* Water is one of *the most important* elements for good health and weight loss. It can suppress the appetite by giving you a feeling of fullness, and it facilitates good colon function and flushes toxins from the body. Drinking a glass of water before a meal can reduce the desire to overeat. Water also helps the body metabolize stored fat. This is the reason nearly every weight-loss program emphasizes that you drink at least 64 ounces of water every day. Herbal teas and diluted juices can be substituted for some of your water quota.

5. *Avoid sweets.* Sugars, natural and refined, are mostly or completely empty calories. They are more likely to get stored as fat than utilized for energy. Also, sweets stimulate the appetite. Artificial sweeteners, like aspartame (NutraSweet), can be worse for appetite stimulation than refined sugar. A study published in 1997 followed 14 dieting women who were given lemonade sweetened with either sucrose (refined sugar) or aspartame (NutraSweet). Both groups ate significantly more when they drank the aspartame-sweetened beverages.

6. *Exercise regularly.* Exercise is essential for weight loss. Aerobic exercise is the only way to burn fat and develop lean body mass. The more muscle you have, the more calories you will burn, even at a resting heart rate. Include aerobic activities three to five times a week: walking, jogging, running, cycling, swimming, aerobic dance, or step aerobics. (See the Exercise and Strength Endurance Section, page 123, for more information.)

NUTRIENT RECOMMENDATIONS

- *Pantothenic acid,* one of the B vitamins, is important in fat metabolism. One study found that individuals taking supplemental pantothenic acid lost weight at an average of 1.2 kg per week. Best juice sources: broccoli, cauliflower, and kale.

- *Chromium* helps the body develop a good insulin response. Insulin plays a critical part in maintaining steady blood sugar levels and in stimulating *thermogenesis* (heat production, which means more calories burned). Chromium can help to increase lean tissue—more muscle means more fat-burning potential. Presumably, this is due to increased insulin sensitivity. In one study, those taking the 200-mcg and the 400-mcg dose of chromium lost an average of 4.2 pounds of fat and gained 1.4 pounds of muscle (versus the placebo group that lost only 0.4 fat pounds and gained only 0.2 pounds in muscle). The recommended daily intake of chromium is between 50 and 200 mcg, yet it appears to be in short supply in the American diet. A USDA study found that nine out of ten adults get less than 50 mcg of chromium daily. Best juice sources: potatoes, green bell peppers, apples, parsnips, spinach, and carrots.

HERBAL RECOMMENDATIONS

Bladder wrack and *hawthorn berries* stimulate the adrenal glands and improve thyroid function.

Chickweed has been used to reduce appetite.

Dandelion, juniper berries, parsley, alfalfa sprouts, and *thyme* have diuretic properties and thus aid in excretion of excess water and detoxification. You can juice alfalfa sprouts, dandelion leaves, and parsley.

Ginger root has thermogenic properties. With some people the tendency to become overweight may be related to a metabolic makeup that results in low thermogenesis. Foods such as ginger root can help facilitate energy production, which may promote weight loss.

JUICE RECOMMENDATIONS

Beet, cabbage, carrot, celery, cucumber, kale, parsley, turnip, spinach, watercress, and wheatgrass. See The Morning Energizer (page 16), Triple C (page 20), Popeye's Power (page 21), and Wheatgrass Light (page 21).

Jerusalem artichoke and parsnip juice can help curb cravings. See The Weight-Loss Buddy (page 29) and Beautiful Skin, Hair, and Nails Cocktail (page 24).

Cucumber, watermelon, parsley, asparagus, lemon, kiwifruit, and cantaloupe (with seeds) are good diuretics. See Weight-Loss Express (page 28), Afternoon Refresher (page 18), Strawberry-Cantaloupe Cocktail (page 38), and Watermelon Refresher (page 40).

Radish juice helps stimulate the thyroid. An efficient thyroid is key to weight loss and maintenance. See Radish Solution, page 30.

Daikon radish has been used in traditional oriental medicine to help eliminate excess fats. See Orient Express, page 18.

1. Sources of pantothenic acid: Beautiful Bone Solution (page 25) and Cherie's Quick-Energy Soup (page 62)

2. Sources of chromium: The Ginger Hopper (page 17), Beautiful Skin, Hair, and Nails Cocktail (page 24), and Bone Power Plus smoothie (page 57)

Try the fizzes (pages 48–53) for refreshing, low-calorie beverages that are actually good for you. With only 5 calories, you can't go wrong with the Skinny Sip, page 50! The following recipes are suggestions for juice combinations using the fruits and vegetables highest in the nutrients recommended for weight loss.

JUICING FOR BABIES AND CHILDREN

RAPID GROWTH AND DEVELOPMENT CHARACTERIZE the first two years of a baby's life. In the first four months, babies will double their weight and triple it by the end of the first year. The foods babies eat in this period of time can affect them for a lifetime. For example, babies that develop iron-deficiency anemia are at a higher risk of experiencing long-term developmental and cognitive problems than babies with normal iron levels.

Infants have unique nutritional needs at the various stages of development. At each level, up to age two, your child's nutritional needs change and must be met for his growing body. Knowing what to juice and how to feed your child can make a big difference in whether he or she is sickly and experiences impaired cognitive functions, or is healthy and capable of learning and doing well in school.

JUICING FOR INFANTS UP TO SIX MONTHS OLD

1. *The only juice your baby should have in the first six months of life is mom's milk.* The American Academy of Pediatrics recommends that infants be breast-fed for the first six to twelve months. The only alternative is iron-fortified infant formula, if you cannot breast-feed. Research shows that infants who are fed breast milk are given a much healthier start, so it is to your baby's advantage if you can breast-feed. No juice or any other food should be given to your baby during this developmental stage, because an infant's gut is very permeable, and large molecules from these foods can be taken up and cause food allergies.

Breast milk contains everything an infant needs and is superior to formula. Its growth factors promote gastrointestinal development and its enzymes facilitate digestion and prevent infections. Formulas have a different whey-to-casein ratio than mother's milk; they contain no growth factors, hormones, or live cells; they lack omega-3 and omega-6 fatty acids; and they provide no protection against infections, allergies, and other diseases. Breast-fed infants have a lower incidence of ear infections, upper respiratory infections, diarrheal gastroenteritis, stomach-flu infections, atopic disease, celiac sprue, Crohn's disease, and insulin-dependent diabetes. Breast-fed babies also have greater acceptance of vegetables and other solid foods, when it is time to introduce these foods, than formula-fed babies. (For more information, see Healthy Breast-feeding, page 150.)

2. *Do not give your baby whole cow's milk before one year of age.* Recent research has shown that iron status is significantly impaired when whole cow's milk is introduced into the diet of six-month-old or younger infants. Also, because the immature gastrointestinal tract is permeable, as mentioned earlier, there is an increased uptake of dietary protein from the intestine, which may contribute to cow's milk protein allergy. This affects 4 to 7.5 percent of the infant population.

3. *Do not microwave or heat breast milk.* A 1992 study shows that microwaving breast milk, even at a low setting, can destroy some of its important disease-fighting capabilities. Breast milk can be refrigerated for days or frozen up to a month, but it should be thawed or warmed only at room temperature. Heating the milk to a body temperature of 37°C can break down antibodies and infection-fighting agents (especially lysozymes, which fight bacteria). Heated breast milk also fosters the growth of more potentially pathogenic bacteria. Breast milk heated to a high setting of 72°C to 98°C in the aforementioned study lost 96 percent of its lysozyme activity and 98 percent of its immunoglobulin-A antibody agents. This study also showed that microwaving itself caused some damage to the breast milk above and beyond the heating.

4. *Drink fresh juices for your baby.* The nutrients will be passed on to your baby through your breast milk. See the section on breast-feeding and juicing, page 150.

JUICING FOR INFANTS SIX MONTHS TO ONE YEAR OLD

1. *Introduce solid food and fresh juice around six months of age.* When a baby is about six months old, it is time to introduce solid food. Feed your baby only one food or juice at a time and try that food for about four days to see if he or she shows any signs of intolerance, such as diarrhea. Usually, the first recommended food is iron-fortified cereal, because a baby's iron stores begin to be depleted about this time. Pureed fruits that are rich in vitamin C, such as orange/pear, cantaloupe, papaya, strawberry, and tangerine/pear are great next additions, because vitamin C increases the absorption of iron, which is difficult to absorb from plant foods. Introduce one fruit at a time, and then combine oranges with pears, for example, when both fruits are tolerable. When you introduce vegetables and their juices, avoid high-oxalate foods the first year; these include spinach, beet greens, chard, and rhubarb. These foods can bind up calcium so that it is not absorbed from that meal. By contrast, kale is a high-calcium food, which can be mixed with a sweet juice such as carrot or pear; always dilute juice with an equal amount of water for babies this age.

2. *Juicing for your baby.*   It is ideal to start with sweeter-tasting juices such as carrot, cantaloupe, or orange, one at a time. Always remove skins, peels, and green tops of carrots for babies. Strain the juice to remove any foam, and *always* dilute the juice with an equal amount of purified water. Purchase organically grown fruits and vegetables whenever possible to avoid pesticides. Apple juice can cause diarrhea for some babies, so watch carefully when it is introduced. Too much fruit juice can spoil your baby's appetite for breast milk or formula, causing him to miss important nutrients for development. Finally, never let your baby suck on a bottle for prolonged periods of time, or go to bed with a bottle of juice in his mouth. The sugars can lead to problems with tooth development and cavities.

3. *Do not feed your baby whole cow's milk up to one year of age.*   The American Academy of Pediatrics states that cow's milk and low-iron formula should not be used in the first year of life. Whole cow's milk has definitely been shown to increase the risk of blood loss, even up to one year of age. One study documented that intestinal blood loss increased by 30 percent in infants fed whole cow's milk. Also, iron deficiency can occur with infants fed whole cow's milk up to one year of age. (For more information, see the section on iron under Healthy Breast-feeding, page 150.)

4. *Never give honey to a baby under one year of age.*   Honey contains bacteria spores that can cause botulism. Though the mature gut of an adult can handle these spores, the gut of a small child under one year of age cannot. This applies to processed as well as raw honey. (Omit honey from all smoothie recipes.)

JUICING FOR CHILDREN ONE TO TWO YEARS OF AGE

By this time your baby's body has matured to the point where the gut is no longer so permeable, and stomach acid is up to normal levels. Now you can introduce other protein foods besides breast milk or formula, and your baby can also enjoy a wider variety of foods and juices. Because your child is now entering a slower growth phase, his appetite will decrease. This is the stage when your infant will play with his food. He will be more interested in the texture and feel of the food and how he eats it than in eating itself.

1. *Feed your child a variety of foods.* You may continue to breast-feed your baby, but it is only one part of his expanding diet. If you choose to give him cow's milk and he shows no signs of intolerance, make sure it is whole milk, not skim or low-fat milk. Toddlers need fat in their diets for growth and development and should be fed a higher-fat diet until age three to four. He can have butter; eggs; cold-pressed or expeller-pressed oils; peanut, almond, and cashew butters; and whole dairy products, if tolerated. Toddlers who are fed a low-fat diet can develop "failure to thrive" syndrome. Avoid "bad fats" such as fried foods, margarine, and fried chips; they are high in trans-fatty acids, which can be carcinogenic (see the section "Fats and Oils" under the Vibrant Health Diet Guidelines, page 177).

Keep in mind that dairy products can cause problems, such as upper respiratory infections, for some children. A large percentage of ear infections are caused by dairy products. The medical director at the clinic where I worked for several years always took children off all dairy products before recommending tubes for their ears. Rice milk or soy milk, fortified with calcium and vitamin D, may be a good alternative.

The healthiest diet for your toddler is organically grown, homemade food. The processing of canned and bottled foods and juices causes many of the nutrients and much of the "life force" to be destroyed. You can buy a food grinder, or puree foods in a blender or food processor; you also can mash vegetables and fruits by hand. Do not add extra salt or sugar to your infant's food—it already contains all the natural sodium and sugars your child needs. If you start out right, your child's taste buds won't demand as much salt or sugar as he or she matures.

2. *Fresh juice should become a regular part of your child's diet.* This is a very good time to give your child two or three glasses of fresh juice a day. Juicing fruits and vegetables makes it easier to feed children more of the nutrients they need for growth. They can have a fruit juice in the morning and one or two vegetable juice combinations in the afternoon or evening. Limit fruit juice to no more than 12 ounces per day (that's before dilution with water). Too much fruit juice has been linked with failure to thrive, short stature, and obesity. Dilute both vegetable and fruit juices with water, but now the ratio can change to one part water for every three parts juice.

Dietary Recommendations

If you are still breast-feeding, your toddler will receive nutrients primarily from you, so following the suggestions in Healthy Breast-feeding (pages 150–152) is important. Children who are no longer breast-feeding should eat a nutrient-rich diet. See the Nutritional Recommendations in the next section—"Juicing for Children Ages Three to Twelve."

Juices for Your Child

Carrot/pear: A rich source of carotenes, trace minerals, and phytonutrients.

Orange/grapefruit: Loaded with vitamin C and bioflavonoids.

Tomato/lemon: Tomatoes are high in lycopene (a carotene with more antioxidant capabilities than beta carotene), and lemons offer vitamin C and bioflavonoids.

Kale/pineapple ($\frac{1}{2}$ kale leaf to 2-inch chunk pineapple): Kale is an excellent source of potassium, calcium, carotenes, iron, and phytonutrients; pineapple offers bromelain, a digestive enzyme. (One cup of kale actually has more calcium than one cup of milk.) See Sweet Calcium Cocktail, page 24.

Watermelon: Contains trace minerals and water; the nutritional quality greatly improves when juiced with the rind and seeds. (See Watermelon Refresher, page 40.)

Pear/peach: Pears are an excellent source of water-soluble fibers and contain trace minerals; soluble fibers are important for intestinal regularity.

JUICING FOR CHILDREN AGES THREE TO TWELVE

This slower growth phase will remain fairly constant until puberty. Now is the time to lower fat intake and teach your child healthy eating habits. Studies show that many diseases such as atherosclerosis begin in childhood. Unfortunately, many children eat large quantities of fat-laden junk food like fried chips and french fries, which can cause fat deposits to begin forming in their arteries. A two-year study by the U.S. Department of Agriculture in 1989 found that nearly one-quarter of all vegetables consumed by children and adolescents were french fries. Only one in five children ate five or more servings of fruits and vegetables per day.

Dietary Recommendations

1. *Serve your child five to nine servings of vegetables and fruits each day.* The USDA Food Guide recommendation is three to five servings of vegetables and two to four servings of fruit each day. Often children say they don't like the taste of vegetables and refuse to eat most of them. Juicing vegetables is one way around this challenge. Tuck some parsley, kale, or a piece of broccoli stem, for example, in a carrot/apple base. (See The Ginger Hopper, page 17, for the recipe; leave out the ginger if your child doesn't like the spicy taste.) A little peanut sauce can go a long way in disguising steamed kale or other vegetables. (I have a recipe for quick peanut sauce in my cookbook *The Healthy Gourmet* [Clarkson Potter, 1996].) You also can add vegetables your child would not otherwise eat to soups and stews. George Foreman told me that is how he grew up big and strong. While searching for the few pieces of meat in his mother's vegetable soups and stews, he was forced to consume a lot of vegetables in the process. (George and I coauthored *Knock-Out-the-Fat Barbecue and Grilling Cookbook* [Villard, 1996].)

2. *Limit fruit juice to no more than 12 ounces per day, and avoid soda pop and powdered drink mixes as much as possible.* Studies indicate that too much fruit juice, soda pop, and Kool-Aid-type drinks have been linked with failure to thrive, short stature, and obesity. It is best to serve fruit juice in small glasses (6 to 8 ounces), dilute it with mineral water or water, or combine it with vegetable juice. Fresh fruit smoothies make a great breakfast-in-a-glass on busy days or a healthy snack after school. (See the smoothie section, pages 54 to 62, for recipe ideas.) Avoid soda pop because it contains phosphates, which bind calcium—a much-needed mineral for forming bones and teeth. Pop also is loaded with chemicals and sugars, either artificial or refined. Diet sodas are usually sweetened with aspartame (NutraSweet). Aspartame contains phenylalanine and aspartic acid. Critics say that high concentrations of phenylalanine can cause mental retardation in some children and aspartic acid in high doses can act as a neurotoxin and promote hormonal disorders (*Nutrition Week,* 1995).* Make your own "pop" with fruit juices and sparkling water (see Fizzes, page 48). Powdered drink mixes like Kool-Aid contain sugar and artificial ingredients. And all these beverages, given in too high a quantity, can spoil your child's appetite for other nutrient-rich foods.

3. *Now is the time to limit fat intake to 25 to 30 percent of your child's calories.* Surveys show that childhood obesity is on the rise. The National Health and Nutrition Examination Survey (NEHANES 3, 1988–1991) shows that four-fifths of the children surveyed, ages 6 to 19, consumed over 30 percent of their calories from fat. Make sure that the largest percentage of fat in your child's diet is not saturated (i.e., from animal sources) and that it is not "bad fat" from fried foods, margarine, fried chips, and hydrogenated oils (they have reached high temperatures in processing). These high-fat foods contain trans-fatty acids, a carcinogenic by-product from oils heated to a high temperature. (For more information on fats and oils, see that section under the Vibrant Health Diet, page 174.)

Nutrient Recommendations

All nutrients are important for your child. I have highlighted here those most crucial for growing children.

- *Vitamin A and provitamin A (carotenes)* strengthen the immune system, improve resistance to infection, especially of the respiratory system, promote healthy cell growth, and are essential for healthy eyes and skin. Carotenes are converted to vitamin A by the body as they are needed. A study in 1931 revealed that schoolchildren who had diets high in carotenes (measured by blood level) missed the fewest number of school days due to illness. Best juice sources: carrots, kale, parsley, spinach, beet greens, chives, mangos, red bell peppers, cantaloupes, apricots, broccoli, romaine lettuce, and papayas.

- *Vitamin C* helps build resistance to infections, helps with physical and mental stress, and is essential for growth and repair of tissues. It

---

*To get a free copy of the four-page FDA report "Summary of Adverse Reactions Attributed to Aspartame," send a self-addressed, stamped envelope to Center for Nutrition Information, 910 17th Street NW, Suite 413, Washington, DC 20006.

increases the absorption of iron when consumed at the same meal. Children often shun vitamin C–rich foods, which are primarily fruits and vegetables. But most children like vegetable-fruit juice combinations, fizzes (fruit juice and sparkling mineral water), and fresh fruit smoothies. Best juice sources: bell peppers, kale, parsley, broccoli, Brussels sprouts, cauliflower, cabbage, strawberries, papayas, spinach, citrus fruits, mangos, and asparagus.

- *Vitamin D* is not really a vitamin; in its active form it is considered a hormone, and our bodies make it from sunlight. It is important for the metabolism of calcium and phosphorus. In children, the classic result of vitamin D deficiency is rickets, which is characterized by stunted growth, delayed tooth development, weakness, and irreversible bone deformities. Best food sources: sardines, salmon, tuna, shrimp, butter, sunflower seeds, eggs, fortified milk and soy milk, mushrooms, and natural cheeses. There are no foods high in vitamin D that can be juiced, except sunflower sprouts.

- *Vitamin B$_6$* is needed for proper growth and maintenance of almost all bodily functions. Babies fed formulas low in vitamin B$_6$ have suffered epileptic-type convulsions, weight loss, nervous irritability, and stomach problems. These problems and other forms of childhood epilepsy respond to vitamin B$_6$ supplementation. Autistic children have improved when given B$_6$ along with magnesium. Best juice sources: kale, bananas, avocados, spinach, potatoes, prunes, and Brussels sprouts. (Bananas and avocados do not juice well, but bananas make great additions to smoothies [pages 54–62] and avocado is delicious in my Quick-Energy Soup, page 62.)

- *Calcium* is necessary for bone and tooth enamel formation as well as for many other important functions of the body. Children up to age 11 need about 800 milligrams of calcium per day; ages 11 to 24 need about 1,200 mg. Best juice sources: kale, parsley, watercress, broccoli, spinach, romaine lettuce, green beans, oranges, celery, and carrots.

- *Zinc* boosts the immune system, is an important factor in wound healing, and is necessary for growth. Studies indicate that children show failure to grow and poor appetite when they are zinc deficient. Best juice sources: ginger root, parsley, potatoes, garlic, carrots, grapes, spinach, cabbage, and cucumbers.

JUICE RECOMMENDATIONS

The following recipes are suggestions for juice combinations using fruits and vegetables highest in the recommended nutrients for children.

1. Sources of carotenes: The Morning Energizer (page 16) and Santa Fe Salsa Cocktail (page 19)

2. Sources of vitamin C and bioflavonoids: Morning Express (page 20) and Morning Sunrise (page 39)

3. Sources of vitamin B_6: Rise and Shake smoothie (page 55), Muscle Power Plus smoothie (page 56), and Cherie's Quick-Energy Soup (page 62)

4. Sources of calcium: Beautiful Bone Solution (page 25), Bone Power Plus (page 57), Sweet Calcium Cocktail (page 24), and The Champ (page 56)

5. Sources of zinc: The Ginger Hopper (page 17), Ginger Waldorf (page 17), and Apple Spice (page 36)

6. For healthy thirst quenchers, choose from the fizzes such as Berry Cool (page 49) and Sparkling Strawberry (page 49). The fizzes are much better for your child than soda pop (loaded with phosphates that bind calcium) or Kool-Aid-type powdered drink mixes (loaded with sugar, dyes, and other additives).

7. Instead of high-fat, high-sugar sweets, try healthy frozen treats from the Freezes section: Strawberry Sorbet (page 64) and Orange, Strawberry, or Peach Creamsicles (page 67)

Note: Watch apple juice for intolerance reactions; apple juice adversely affects some children.

HEALTHY PREGNANCY

GOOD NUTRITION BEFORE AND DURING pregnancy can have a very positive long-term effect for both you and your baby. Getting the right nutrients is considered one of *the most important* factors in influencing fetal development and an uncomplicated delivery. Surveys show that a significant number of U.S. women of childbearing age consume diets that are inadequate in certain nutrients associated with a healthy pregnancy, such as zinc, folic acid, vitamin B_6, iron, and calcium.

During pregnancy, many physiological adjustments are taking place in your body to accommodate the growth and development of the fetus. These changes will cause an average weight gain of 20 percent, which is due to conceptus (placenta, fetus, and amniotic fluid) and maternal components (uterine changes, breast growth, fat storage, and increased extracellular fluid). All these changes promote growth of the fetus and prepare your body for delivery and lactation.

DIETARY RECOMMENDATIONS

If you are considering pregnancy, start immediately to prepare your body nutritionally for the demands pregnancy will make. The early weeks of gestation are a crucial period of fetal development; this is not a time to fall short on nutrients. If you are pregnant, make healthy eating your top priority, and include a wide variety of whole foods (unrefined) in your diet. Also, by eating a balanced diet and drinking nutrient-rich juices, you will receive even greater benefit from your prenatal vitamins.

1. *Protein* is necessary for the growth of the fetus, placenta, uterus, breasts, and blood cells, as well for as milk production. Eating too little protein during pregnancy can adversely affect the development of your baby. For example, infant brain growth can be stunted by protein deficiency. Best food sources: organically grown, lean red meat (also the best source of iron and vitamin B_{12}), poultry, fish, eggs, dairy products, or legumes (beans, lentils, split peas), combined with whole grains, nuts, seeds, and soy products such as tofu and tempeh.

2. *Complex carbohydrates* provide energy fuel. For more information on the type of carbohydrates to choose, see Basic Guidelines for the Vibrant Health Diet, page 174.

3. *Good fats* provide fat-soluble vitamins, are an important source of energy, and are essential components of cell membranes and the central nervous system. The fats you choose are crucial. For example, docosahexaenoic acid (DHA), found in fish oils, is necessary for brain and eye development. Deficiencies during pregnancy can lead to permanent learning disabilities and a decrease in visual acuity in the fetus. See recommendation for "Fats and Oils" under Basic Dietary Guidelines in the Vibrant Health Diet, page 177.

4. *Juice, juice, juice!* Emphasis should be placed on improving the nutritional quality of your diet rather than on eating more food. The addition of vegetable and fruit juices is an easy way to get concentrated nutrients without excess calories. Many nutrients work together in your body, and fresh juice will supply nutritional compounds that are not in your vitamin/mineral supplements. Keep in mind that many phytonutrients, enzymes, soluble fiber, and other compounds are not available in supplemental form—some have probably not yet been discovered; nevertheless, they are all needed to work together biochemically in your body. This is one of the best times to keep your juicer running and drink your vitamin-mineral cocktails daily. (Do not juice-fast while you are pregnant.)

5. *Choose organically grown food; reduce exposure to toxins.* It is important to eliminate potentially toxic substances. Exposure to toxins in utero through maternal consumption of contaminated foods affects memory and learning abilities in children. For example, PCBs have been associated with poorer short-term memory function on both verbal and quantitative tests. Pesticide-sprayed vegetables, fruits, and grains, and animals raised with pesticides, hormones, and antibiotics contribute to toxicity in your system and can potentially interfere with the growth and development of the fetus. Toxic substances such as nitrates increase the risk for childhood nervous system tumors and brain tumors associated with exposure to nitrosamine compounds. See the section Organically Grown, page 180.

NUTRIENT RECOMMENDATIONS

- *Choline* is essential in the development of the brain, and maternal intake can influence memory performance in offspring. Best juice sources: green beans, cabbage, spinach, and oranges.

- *Folic acid* is necessary to prevent neural tube defects such as spina bifida (open spine) and anencephaly (lack of brain). Damage to the spinal cord often keeps children in wheelchairs or on crutches. A landmark study conducted in several countries showed that folic acid prevented 72 percent of neural tube defects. Since this birth defect occurs in the first 28 days after conception, 400 mcg of folic acid daily is recommended for all women capable of getting pregnant. Other studies have shown that women who supplement their diets with vitamins containing folic acid have a reduced chance of bearing an infant with facial clefts (harelip), cardiovascular defects, and urinary tract abnormalities. Folic acid supplementation also decreases the risk for preterm delivery and low-birth-weight infants. Best juice sources: asparagus, spinach, kale, beet greens, broccoli, Brussels sprouts, cabbage, blackberries, and oranges.

- *Vitamin B_6 (pyridoxine)* is of special concern for pregnant and breast-feeding women; studies show that although requirements go up at these times, women may not be getting enough of this vitamin. One study found that during the last month of pregnancy women consumed only 50 percent of the recommended dietary allowance (RDA) for vitamin B_6, and lactating women consumed only 60 percent of the RDA after delivery. Vitamin B_6 has been shown to decrease nausea and vomiting during the first trimester of pregnancy (25 mg three times a day). One study found that Apgar scores were significantly higher for infants of mothers who consumed several times the RDA of B_6 than for those of mothers who took close to the RDA. (Apgar scores evaluate the health and well-being of newborns.) Best juice sources: kale, spinach, turnip greens, bell peppers, Brussels sprouts, bananas, and avocados. (Bananas and avocados do not juice well, but bananas make a great addition to smoothies [see pages 54–62], and avocados make a good base for my Quick-Energy Soup, page 62.)

- *Vitamin D* helps calcium absorption. The body can make vitamin D from sunlight. However, if you live in a primarily overcast climate such as the Pacific Northwest or if you are pregnant during the dark days of winter, it is advisable to supplement your diet with vitamin D–rich foods (e.g., salmon, tuna, sardines, shrimp, sunflower seeds, eggs, mushrooms, natural cheeses, and fortified milk or fortified soy milk). Vitamin D is not available in appreciable amounts in foods that can be juiced, except for sunflower sprouts.

- *Calcium* requirements increase during pregnancy. Between 50 and 350 mg is transferred from the mother's blood supply to the fetus daily. If dietary calcium is not sufficient to meet the needs of the fetus, calcium is taken from the mother's bones. The RDA for calcium during pregnancy is 1,200 mg. Best juice sources: collard and turnip greens, parsley, dandelion greens, watercress, beet greens, broccoli, spinach, romaine lettuce, and green beans.

- *Iron* deficiency is common among pregnant women. Demands for iron increase during the second half of pregnancy. If adequate iron is not supplied, anemia can result. Also, additional iron is needed because of blood loss during delivery. Foods and juices rich in vitamin C, such as leafy greens, citrus fruits, strawberries, papayas, and cantaloupes, enhance the absorption of iron. Best juice sources: parsley, beet greens, dandelion greens, spinach, Jerusalem artichokes, chard, broccoli, cauliflower, strawberries, blackberries, asparagus, and red cabbage.

- *Zinc* is necessary for normal fetal development. It promotes growth of tissues and bones and is involved in making genetic material. Zinc deficiency can cause low birth weight, premature births, and increased complications during pregnancy. Zinc is needed during fetal brain development, and a deficiency can cause brain damage. Best juice sources: ginger root, turnips, parsley, garlic, carrots, grapes, spinach, and cabbage.

HERBAL RECOMMENDATIONS

Ginger root makes a delicious complement to fresh juices, and studies show it can be beneficial in helping decrease the nausea and vomiting associated with morning sickness. Historically, ginger's use has been involved in helping complaints associated with the gastrointestinal tract. It promotes elimination of gas and soothes the intestines. It has been used to treat hyperemesis gravidarum, the most severe form of morning sickness, which usually requires hospitalization.

JUICE RECOMMENDATIONS

Ginger root: The Ginger Hopper (page 17), Ginger Twist (page 17), and Apple Spice (page 36)

The following recipes are suggestions for juice combinations using the fruits and vegetables highest in the recommended nutrients for a healthy pregnancy.

1. Sources of choline: Memory Mender (page 27), Triple C (page 20), and Rise 'n' Shake smoothie—add lecithin granules for an extra helping of choline (page 55)

2. Sources of folic acid: Popeye's Power (page 21), Beautiful Bone Solutions (page 25), and Berry Smooth smoothie—yogurt or soy milk can be substituted for the cashews (page 58)

3. Sources of vitamin B_6: Popeye's Power (page 21), Beautiful Skin, Hair, and Nails Cocktail (page 24), and Jack and the Bean (page 31)

4. Sources of vitamin D: Pure Green Sprout Drink (page 22)

5. Sources of calcium: Beautiful Bone Solution (page 25), Liver Life Cocktail (page 33), and The Champ smoothie (page 56)

6. Sources of iron: Weight-Loss Buddy (page 29), Sweet Dreams Nightcap (page 29), and Berry Smooth smoothie (page 58)

7. Sources of zinc: The Morning Energizer (page 16), The Ginger Hopper (page 17), The Immune Builder (page 31), and Grape Expectations (page 40)

HEALTHY BREAST-FEEDING

WHEN YOU ARE BREAST-FEEDING, your diet is just as important as when you are pregnant. The nutrients your baby did not or could not store before birth must be supplied through breast milk. All nutrients are important, but I have highlighted those you should especially focus on.

DIETARY RECOMMENDATIONS

1. *Calories/energy.*   You need more energy now than during pregnancy. About 500 extra calories per day are required for producing milk. In the first three months, 150 to 300 calories can come from the fat stored during pregnancy; after that, it must come from food.

2. *Protein.*   Breast-feeding requires more protein than pregnancy—an additional 15 grams daily for the first six months and 12 grams daily for the next six months. Sprouts are an additional source of amino acids, and they can be juiced. (See Pure Green Sprout Drink, page 22.)

3. *Juices.*   Your body will draw from its stores of nutrients to produce milk; however this has limits, especially concerning water-soluble vitamins, which are typically found in low levels in human milk if the mother's diet is low in these nutrients. Poor nutrition can also cause low milk production. For these reasons, it is recommended that you not diet while breast-feeding and that you consume 3 to 4 quarts of liquid per day. This is why juicing makes perfect sense. Juices are low in calories, high in nutrients (especially the water-soluble vitamins you need to replenish continually—vitamin C and the B vitamins), and packed with water. Fresh juices supply you, and therefore your baby through your breast milk, with an abundance of vitamins, minerals, enzymes, phytonutrients, soluble fibers, and that special life force, which is energy converted from the sun through photosynthesis into vibrating energy that is passed on to our bodies when we eat and juice the plants. Harry Oldfield has photographed breast milk and formula (in a process known as *kirlian photography*) to capture their energy fields. In *The Dark Side of the Brain* (Element, 1991), Oldfield printed a picture of breast milk, showing luminous rays of vibrating light, and one of formula, which emitted no light rays. One can conclude that if a breast-feeding mother consumes more high-energy foods, these subtle energies are passed on to her baby in breast milk. (For more information on the benefits of juice and raw food, and for an explanation of kirlian photography, see Basic Guidelines for the Vibrant Health Diet, page 177.)

NUTRIENT RECOMMENDATIONS

- *Vitamin B$_6$* is especially important to lactating women. Studies have shown the requirements for this vitamin go up during breast-feeding. Vitamin B$_6$ is of special concern not only for you but for your infant. One study found that Apgar scores were significantly higher for infants of mothers who consumed several times the B$_6$ RDA than for those of mothers who took close to the RDA. (Apgar scores, taken on newborns, are predictors of general health and well-being.) B$_6$ is important during lactation because B$_6$ deficiency is associated with convulsions and irritability in some infants. Best juice sources: bananas, avocados, kale, spinach, turnip greens, bell peppers, potatoes, prunes, and Brussels sprouts. (Bananas and avocados do not juice well, but bananas make great additions to smoothies, pages 54–62, and avocado is a part of my Quick-Energy Soup, page 62.)

- *Vitamin D* deficiency causes rickets in infants; it is characterized by a softened skull. Vitamin D deficiency can lead to bone deformities, stunted growth, weakness, and delayed tooth development. Vitamin D is not truly a vitamin but a hormone in its active form; it is made by our bodies from sunlight. In the dark days of winter or if you live in a largely overcast climate like the Pacific Northwest, make sure you eat plenty of vitamin D–rich foods. Best food sources: sardines, salmon, tuna, shrimp, butter, sunflower seeds, eggs, fortified milk and soy milk, mushrooms, and natural cheeses. Foods that can be juiced are not high in vitamin D, except for sunflower sprouts.

- *Calcium* intake should be 1,200 milligrams daily during lactation. If you do not ingest adequate calcium, your body will leach it from your bones. Low calcium intake is clearly a major factor in the development of osteoporosis. Best juice sources: kale, dandelion greens, watercress, beet greens, broccoli, spinach, romaine lettuce, green beans, oranges, celery, and carrots.

- *Iron*. According to the American Academy of Pediatrics, iron deficiency in early childhood may lead to long-term changes in behavior that may not be reversible with iron supplementation, even though the anemia is corrected. Best juice sources: parsley, Jerusalem artichokes, broccoli, cauliflower, strawberries, and asparagus.

- *Zinc* is very important for growth. Low zinc levels have been associated with low birth weight, failure to thrive, impaired glucose tolerance, and increased incidence of schizophrenia. Best juice sources: ginger root, turnips, parsley, potatoes, garlic, and carrots.

HERBAL RECOMMENDATIONS

Garlic was found in one study to enhance breast-feeding. It was noted in this study that the odor of the breast milk was stronger, and the infants liked it as evidenced by sucking longer and consuming more milk.

JUICE RECOMMENDATIONS

The following recipes are suggestions for juice combinations using the fruits and vegetables highest in the recommended nutrients for lactation.

1. Sources of vitamin B₆: Rise and Shake smoothie (page 55), Mango Mania smoothie (page 57), and Cherie's Quick-Energy Soup (page 62)

2. Sources of vitamin D: Pure Green Sprout Drink (page 22)

3. Sources of calcium: The Morning Energizer (page 16), Beautiful Bone Solution (page 25), and The Champ smoothie (page 56)

4. Sources of iron: The Memory Mender (page 27), Spring Tonic (page 33), and Strawberry-Cantaloupe Cocktail (page 38)

5. Sources of zinc: The Ginger Hopper (page 17), Ginger Twist (page 17), and Apple Spice (page 36)

6. Good supply of extra calories for energy: The Champ smoothie (page 56) and Cherie's Quick-Energy Soup (page 62)

JUICY TIPS
FOR PETS

DECADES AGO FAMILY PETS WERE fed only table scraps. That is all there was. Most animals ate vegetables from the garden (grown naturally without pesticides or chemical fertilizers), whole grains, and leftover meat or poultry.

Today, the pet food market is an $8 billion industry. The majority of commercial dog and cat foods, either canned products or bagged dry foods, are processed at high temperatures—above 212°F. This high heat destroys enzymes and naturally occurring vitamins; in other words, the life force of the food is gone. High heat also breaks down major nutrient groups of proteins, fats, and carbohydrates into fragments that become difficult to digest and may even have a toxic effect on a pet's immune system.

Pet food protein sources—usually chicken, beef, or lamb—are purchased from mass producers. Most of these animals have been raised on hormones, antibiotics, and other drugs and have not been fed an organically grown diet. Additives and preservatives are added to many brands of pet food. Furthermore, most of the animal products have been rejected for human consumption and classified as "4D"—meats derived from dying, diseased, or disabled animals. Protein sources may contain other undigestible materials and by-products such as feathers, beaks, cartilage, and lung material. They often contain grain by-products that have been grown with chemical fertilizers and sprayed with pesticides.

There is a strong link between poor-quality ingredients and the widespread health problems in our pets. Is it any wonder that our little buddies are slowly starving for the life force that only fresh, whole foods can provide?

What can you do when you are too busy to make homemade dinners for your animal? The answer is to feed your furry friend(s) life-giving, nutrient-rich juices every day. Our schnauzer, MacKenzie, won't drink a bowl of carrot juice, so we add several tablespoons of juice to his wet food along with chopped veggies, olive oil, and pulp from juicing (see Basic Healthy Recipe that follows). He loves his "gourmet dinners." If your cat or dog won't lap up fresh juice, try our recipe.

BASIC HEALTHY RECIPE

Mix one or two tablespoons of carrot juice or a combination of vegetable-fruit juices (no citrus or tomato; it's too acidic for animals) with some of your pet's wet food, and stir in a tablespoon or two of leftover pulp from juicing (organic is best; it's believed more pesticides cling to the fiber). Add a tablespoon of finely chopped, raw vegetables such as broccoli or cauliflower and some leftover brown rice, millet, or oatmeal. Leftover steamed vegetables or a portion of a baked potato also make a good addition. Drizzle a little olive oil ($\frac{1}{2}$ to 1 teaspoon) on top and you'll have a power meal that will boost your pet's health. Add an extra serving or two per week of chicken, lamb, beef, tofu, or egg yolk—raised organically and antibiotic-free and hormone-free. These proportions are for a medium-size dog (15 to 35 pounds).

It also helps to choose a very good brand of canned pet food that has no preservatives. For a natural-pet-food rating of canned foods, get the February 1998 issue of Dr. Bob and Susan Goldstein's newsletter "Love of Animals" (800-711-2292). I switched recently to Lick Your Chops brand for MacKenzie, at the Goldsteins' recommendation, and he is feeling better than ever! You may want to subscribe to their newsletter, as we do, and get a whopping supply of healthy pet advice.

Try some of the following juice combinations for your pet, and be sure to make some extra for yourself at the same time.

JUICE RECOMMENDATIONS TO KEEP YOUR PET HEALTHY

- *Carrot/celery:* Carrots are rich in beta carotene, a powerful antioxidant. The enzymes in carrots are most effective when the carrot is juiced. Enzymes help the intestines break down and absorb the nutrients in food. Once the nutrients are absorbed into the bloodstream, they can get into cells and tissues to help rebuild internal organs and revitalize the body. Celery is one of the best sources of organic sodium. Organic sodium acts very differently in the body than sodium chloride; it feeds cells, whereas sodium chloride (table salt) is difficult to digest and can cause water retention. Without an abundance of raw food, most animals are very deficient in organic sodium.

- *Green drink:* Use parsley, watercress, spinach, wheatgrass, sprouts, or kale, mixed with carrot. Green juices are good tonics for the immune system and are excellent blood purifiers.

- *Grape:* Grapes are a source of anthocyanidins and proanthocyanidins, a class of water-soluble bioflavonoids known as *polyphenols.* Members of this class of bioflavonoids are very powerful antioxidants. They are quickly absorbed and remain at the cellular level for up to 48 hours. You've no doubt heard of grape seed extract, which can be purchased in supplement form. Juice your grapes with seeds, and you'll have your own inexpensive form, but be sure to choose organically grown grapes, as pesticide sprays tend to seep easily into the thin skins of the grapes.

- *Asparagus:* Add a tablespoon or two of fresh asparagus juice to your pet's water or wet food. It's a powerful, natural diuretic and will help your pet lose weight and cleanse the kidneys. This also can energize older animals that may be retaining water. Remain attentive after your pet drinks this juice, however, as he or she may need to go outside or to the litter box more than once in the hours that follow.

- *Melon or cucumber:* Melon and cucumber juices are also good diuretics.

Reminder: Don't feed citrus or tomato juices to your pets; they are too acidic for animals.

HEALING PETS WITH FRESH JUICE

Never underestimate the healing power of nutrition when your pet is ill. "Power Cocktails" and nutrient-rich foods can boost a flagging immune system. Live-food juices provide digestible amino acids, which the body uses to manufacture more immunoproteins—necessary to fight disease and injury. While the juice remedies go to work delivering their healing powers to weak areas of the body, the enzymes, vitamins, minerals, and phytonutrients cleanse and restore the body.

Animals do their own juicing in nature. Have you ever watched your dog or cat munch on grass? She is making her own "green drink," which detoxifies and rejuvenates her body. Sometimes your pet will regurgitate the fibrous grass as it purges the system. Don't be alarmed when this happens or deny your pet this life-giving food. However, juicing greens is much better for your pet—it's easier to digest and more easily absorbed.

If your pet is ill, please read the story "Brunzi's Best," page 195. I cried when I heard Carol's account of her beloved golden retriever's diagnosis of cancer and his recovery. I think Brunzi's story will inspire you to change your pet's diet so he or she can have the best chance for recovery.

NUTRIENT RECOMMENDATIONS

Clinical veterinary nutrition research provides the following information:

- *Vitamin A* and *provitamin A (carotenes)* increase resistance to infections. Best juice sources: carrots, kale, sweet potatoes, parsley, spinach, beet greens, watercress, and squash.

- *Vitamin E* can enhance immune functions such as cell-mediated immunity (immune mechanisms not controlled by antibodies) and phagocytosis (bacteria digestion). It can also reduce the effects of stress on the immune system. Best juice sources: spinach, asparagus, and carrots.

- *Copper* deficiency can lead to susceptibility to infections due to reduced immune functions. Best juice sources: carrots, garlic, ginger, turnips, and apples.

- *Zinc* supports the thymus gland and cell-mediated immunity. Best juice sources: ginger, parsley, potatoes, garlic, carrots, grapes, spinach, cabbage, lettuce, and cucumbers.

JUICE RECOMMENDATIONS

Choose organic produce whenever possible. See the section Organically Grown for more information, page 180.

The Goldsteins' Instant Immune-Booster Cocktail

2 carrots
2 stalks celery
1 apple
1 handful parsley
1 garlic clove or $1/4$-inch piece ginger
$1/4$ green pepper

Juice all the ingredients, stir to combine, and offer the juice to your pet in a bowl or mix some with his or her wet food.

The Power Cocktail

$1/2$ cup carrot juice
1 tablespoon parsley juice
2 organic egg yolks (no whites)

Place all the ingredients in a blender and combine them on low speed.
   Mix this cocktail with the Basic Healthy Recipe, page 154, as follows:

For cats and small dogs (up to 14 pounds): 2 to 3 tablespoons two to three
   times a day
Medium dogs (15 to 35 pounds): 3 tablespoons two to three times a day
Large dogs (36 to 85 pounds): 3 tablespoons four to six times per day
Extra-large dogs (over 85 pounds): 4 tablespoons four to six times per day

Home Juice Healer
(Adapted from "Love of Animals," April 1998)

Condition	Juice Remedies (organic is best)
Allergies	Kale, parsley, spinach, carrot, and apple
Arthritis	Broccoli, celery, carrot, apple, and ginger
Cancer	Carrot, grape, broccoli, cauliflower, and wheatgrass
Heart disease	Spinach, asparagus, carrot, and apple
Kidney	Asparagus, parsley, cucumber, carrot, and celery
Liver	Dark green lettuce, carrot, beet, cucumber
LUTD*	Asparagus, collard greens, cranberry, apple, and carrot
Obesity	Cucumber, melon, parsley, asparagus, apple, and carrot
Periodontal	Cabbage, beet greens and root, carrot, ginger, and apple

*Lower urinary tract disease.

CLEANSING PROGRAMS

JUST AS A HOME NEEDS a thorough spring cleaning, your body also needs thorough cleansing occasionally, if you want to achieve optimum health. If you take personal hygiene seriously, you may assume that the inside of your body is just as clean as the outside, but given our modern lifestyles, this no longer happens automatically.

The body was set up to handle an occasional toxic substance, such as spoiled food, but not the kind of abuse we encounter as a result of environmental toxins. We are continually seduced by a host of unhealthy substances such as fried foods, high-fat snacks, refined foods, fake foods, and foods with preservatives and dyes. We are bombarded with pesticides, herbicides, chemical fertilizers, and noxious chemicals in our air, soil, and water. All these substances serve to weaken and congest the body.

These toxic and congestive substances can also overwhelm our organs of elimination. Substances that are not broken down and excreted are stored in the liver, kidneys, colon, gallbladder, fat cells, bones, and tissue spaces.

The liver is a prime place to store poisons that can't get excreted. Highly toxic chemicals are known to pass through the liver; they include polycyclic hydrocarbons that make up pesticides and herbicides such as DDT, dioxin, PCB, and PCP. High amounts of these toxins have been found in people's livers. A weakened liver can lead to reduced production of bile acids. Bile ensures that cholesterol stays soluble and does not turn to stones in the gallbladder. When the liver cuts back on bile acid production, either because of its weakened condition, yo-yo dieting, or disease, cholesterol goes unchecked and can form gallstones. Toxins settle in the kidneys, too, causing weakness, sluggishness, and poor performance. The colon can become congested, and as a result will absorb fewer nutrients; it will also leak toxins back into the bloodstream. The skin, which plays a major role in excretion, can become clogged.

It is advantageous to cleanse the various organs of our bodies periodically to promote health and healing. I've learned through personal experience this can happen only through specific plans designed to promote "housecleaning" in each organ.

Detoxifying the body is worth the effort because the benefits are astounding. You will look more vibrant—wrinkles will diminish, skin color will improve, dark circles under the eyes will eventually disappear, and your hair and nails will grow better. Best of all, you will enjoy new health and vitality. You will feel more energetic, have greater mental clarity, and enjoy a greater sense of well-being.

Organically grown, freshly made fruit and vegetable juices will help you no matter what else you do, but with congested organs of elimination, you won't get the best results for all your juicing efforts. It is a bit like continuing to wax a linoleum floor that has old wax and dirt buildup. You will never achieve the clean, shiny floor you want until you first strip off the old gunk. As with the floor, we all need to get rid of the "old gunk" that builds up in our bodies.

What follows are programs for purifying the liver, gallbladder, kidneys, colon, skin, and blood. They work. I urge you to use these cleansing plans periodically because this is one of the most important steps you can take toward improved health and toward getting the full benefit of your juicing for high-level wellness and vibrant good looks.

JUICE FASTING

Every year my husband and I make our annual pilgrimage to the Optimum Health Institute (OHI) of San Diego. We have been going there since 1991 for the cleansing benefits of their weekly raw food and juice fasting program. We call it our "tune-up." We lose weight. Facial lines fade—we both swear the program wipes away at least five years from our faces. (We should go more often or better yet start our own spa!) We always leave feeling renewed. But most important, we will never know the diseases these total body cleansing weeks help us prevent.

No one has been able to explain why drinking only fresh juices for a period of several days works such a miracle, but "miracle" is the right word. Lines on the face soften, the body firms, and the skin and hair look healthier. High blood pressure and cholesterol levels come down. Aches and pains diminish.

Whenever you are sick, the body is sending a signal. It needs rest—both from strenuous work and from foods that are toxic or difficult to digest. Juice fasting gives the digestive system time out. It aids the immune system in clearing out dead, diseased, and damaged cells and supports immune cells with an abundance of nutrients. Sludge that accumulates in interstitial spaces can be cleared away. There is an opportunity to reduce lipofuscin—the brown slime caused by lipid peroxidation that is responsible for age spots. Juice fasting clears out poisons right down to the cellular level.

Juice fasting is a safe and easy way to detoxify your internal organs, tissues, and cells. Fasting has been written about for centuries. It was used by the Essenes, a monastic sect at the time of Christ, and has been a part of nearly all religious practices throughout history. Today the Orthodox Christian Church—Greek, Russian, and Antiochian—carries on the ancient tradition by practicing cycles of fasting and feasting throughout the year.

I do not recommend strict water fasts because they are too hard on the body. Too many toxins are released, and without the addition of nutrients that neutralize and bind them, you can do yourself more harm than good. The antioxidants—vitamins C and E, beta carotene, selenium, and various enzymes and phytochemicals—are in abundance in fresh juices. These scavengers bind harmful toxins and carry them out of the body while you fast.

Some words of caution: Children under 18 should not follow a strict juice fast unless recommended by a health professional; however, fresh fruit and vegetable juices are a great supplement to a child's diet. Diabetics should seek a physician's approval before juice-fasting. Anyone with hypoglycemia should avoid fruit juice and should dilute carrot juice with an equal amount of purified water; the addition of protein powder is also beneficial.

Herbal Recommendations

Beneficial herbal teas: Dandelion root and nettles teas help cleanse the liver and kidneys. (If purchased in bulk, steep ½ teaspoon of either herb in a pint of water, strain, and drink warm. Lemon may be added for flavor.)

Bulking agents such as psyllium husks can be added to fresh juice. They are used as mucilaginous bulk laxatives. Mix two teaspoons to a glass of juice two to three times during the day. These high-fiber agents also help to curb appetite. (For more information, see The Intestinal Cleanse, page 163.)

Juice Recommendations

Cleansing juices: Beets (good for the liver), cabbage, wheatgrass, sprouts, lemon, carrot, celery, green pepper, orange, parsley, grapefruit, and apple
Diuretics: Cucumber, parsley, asparagus, lemon, kiwifruit, watermelon, and cantaloupe with the seeds

The Juice Fast Sample Menu

The suggested menu is a guideline for the juice fast and can be modified whenever necessary to meet your individual needs. The juice recipes are only suggestions; choose any juice recipes you would like any time of day, but do strive for variety, rather than relying on just one or two recipes that are your favorites in order to ensure that you get a range of nutrients. Follow the menu for one to three days.

Breakfast

The Morning Energizer (page 16), Morning Express (page 20), or Magnesium Special (page 22)

Midmorning Break

Waldorf Twist (page 16), The Gallbladder Cleansing Cocktail (page 27), or Digestive Tonic (page 26)

Lunch

Liver Life Tonic, Popeye's Power (page 21) or Cherie's Quick-Energy Soup (page 62)

Happy Hour

Santa Fe Salsa Cocktail (page 19) or Afternoon Refresher (page 18)

Dinner

Spring Tonic (page 33), The Colon Cleanser (page 26), or Pure Green Sprout Drink (page 22)

Bedtime Snack

Sweet Dreams Nightcap (page 29) or Skinny Sip (page 50)

Breaking the Fast

Breaking the fast properly is as important as the fast itself. If the fast is broken with bad food, you could do more harm than good. Eat only vegan food (no animal products) the day after, and eat the largest portion of your food raw—fresh fruits and vegetables. A suggested menu for breaking the juice fast follows. A blank space indicates when you may select the juice or smoothie recipe of your choice.

Breakfast

Juice or smoothie: _____
Fruit or vegetable salad flavored with lemon juice
Herbal tea

Midmorning Snack

Juice: _____

Lunch

Energy Soup (page 62) or any vegetarian soup of your choice
Vegetable salad with lemon juice

Midafternoon Snack

Juice: _____
or herbal tea

Dinner

Vegetable soup or steamed vegetables
Vegetable salad

Bedtime Snack

Vegetable juice: _____
or herbal tea

THE INTESTINAL CLEANSE

The small intestine is made up of three segments: duodenum, jejunum, and ileum. Mineral absorption takes place in the duodenum, the first segment. Absorption of water-soluble vitamins, carbohydrates, and proteins occurs mostly in the jejunum, and the ileum is where fat-soluble vitamins, fat, cholesterol, and bile salts are absorbed. The large intestine (colon) also is made up of three segments: ascending, transverse, and descending colon. The large intestine is where feces are formed. Although most of the water is absorbed from the small intestine, water and electrolytes are absorbed here.

Eating overly cooked food, fried food, junk food, spoiled food, sweets like candy and ice cream, drinking coffee and alcohol, and taking drugs (prescription or recreational) can stimulate the secretion of mucus throughout the entire alimentary canal. The body's natural protective system is equipped to deal with occasional bad food. But when we ingest these substances every day, and for some people at every meal and between meals, the mucus and waste build up in the small intestine and colon.

As intestinal waste accumulates, peristaltic action becomes less effective, and the transit time of material passing through the intestinal tract slows down. This can contribute to constipation and weight gain, which can be exacerbated by a low-fiber diet and not drinking enough water. Mucoid matter and waste buildup can also be a breeding ground for parasites. I struggled with parasites for years until I discovered a more thorough intestinal cleansing process.

Waste buildup in the intestines can also interfere with nutrient absorption, which takes place in the small intestine. Cleansing the entire intestinal tract is an important health measure to enable efficient nutrient absorption into the bloodstream and to reduce toxin reabsorption.

The Intestinal Cleanse Program

1. *Drink three high-fiber "shakes" per day for three to four weeks.* Use psyllium husk and bentonite clay (available at most health food stores) to make your shakes. Psyllium husk powder is a fibrous bulking agent that thickens and gels when mixed with water or juice. Bentonite clay is an absorptive clay, used for centuries for internal purification. It draws out metals, drugs, toxins, waste, and mucus.

Mix 1 tablespoon bentonite clay with 8 to 10 ounces of water or your favorite juice in a jar and shake. Add 2 teaspoons psyllium husk powder and shake again. Drink immediately, as psyllium husk gels quickly and the mixture becomes very thick.

Drink the high-fiber shake for breakfast, midmorning break, and midafternoon. Drink the shakes each day for three to four weeks. The fiber shakes are very filling, and you probably won't be as hungry during this cleanse, which makes it easier to lose weight, if that is a goal. Also, moving fat and cholesterol through the ileum at a healthy pace, thus minimizing their absorption, also facilitates weight loss and weight maintenance. Colonics or enemas greatly facilitate removing excess waste that has accumulated. This also will help relieve any adverse symptoms you may experience as toxins are being released, such as headaches, fatigue, sleepiness, or aches and pains.

2. *Eat two meals a day, making the high-fiber shake and fresh juice your breakfast.* The program works best if both meals are mostly vegetarian (no animal products).

Arise and Shine offers a 10-item colon cleanse program that includes bentonite clay and psyllium husk powder along with two herbal supplements that help clear out colon waste. You can order "Cleanse Thyself Program" at 800-688-2444.

THE GALLBLADDER CLEANSE

The function of the gallbladder is to store and concentrate bile until it is needed in the small intestine. The liver makes bile from the breakdown products of metabolism. Bile acids are the checks and balances of the body, designed to keep cholesterol soluble so it doesn't turn to stones. Stones form when there is an increase in cholesterol or a decrease in bile acids, lecithin, and/or water. The majority of stones found in the U.S. population are a mixture of cholesterol, bile salts, bile pigments, and inorganic salts of calcium. The typical Western diet of high-fat, fiber-depleted, refined foods precipitates gallstones.

Symptoms of gallbladder problems include: Abdominal pain with irregular pain-free intervals of days or months, bloating, gas, nausea, and discomfort after a heavy meal of rich, fatty foods. (Note: Some people with gallbladder problems have no symptoms.)

I did a gallbladder flush for the first time when I was 30 because a reflexologist suggested the program. I experienced considerable pain when he worked on the reflex points on my feet that corresponded with the liver/gallbladder area of my body. I was surprised by the efficacy of the purge, and I've been a believer in this program ever since.

The 7-Day Gallbladder Flush

Monday through Friday, drink at least two 8-ounce glasses of freshly made apple juice. (Choose any apples you wish, such as Golden or Red Delicious, Granny Smith, or pippin.) If you have a sugar metabolism challenge such as hypoglycemia, diabetes, or candidiasis, dilute the apple juice with at least 4 ounces of purified water, or substitute lemon and water. Eat a low-fat, high-fiber diet. Avoid coffee, alcohol, soft drinks, junk food, sweets, meat, dairy, and wheat. Drink only freshly made vegetable and fruit juices on Saturday and eat no solid food. (This is a juice fast day. See page 160 for a sample menu.) Saturday evening before retiring, drink 4 ounces of gently warmed extra-virgin, cold-pressed olive oil mixed with 4 ounces of freshly squeezed lemon juice; shake the mixture in a jar to combine. (This is about the worst stuff I've ever tasted, but it works.) Sunday morning drink 8 ounces of prune juice. Dilute the prune juice with 4 ounces of purified water if you have a sugar metabolism problem. Within a few hours, the gallbladder should purge.

What to expect? Stones can be as small as orange seeds or the size of dimes, or they can appear as a thick liquid if they have been softened by the juices. Colors range from light to dark green to turquoise. (I mention this so you won't think you are viewing something from Mars when the flush is successful.)

Consult your health care professional before trying this program. Also, if you know you have gallstones, suspect that you might, are over 40, or have not experienced cleansing programs before, and you've eaten a typical Western diet most of your life, it's advisable not to try The Gallbladder Flush until you've done several other cleansing programs, including The Liver Cleanse Program and The Intestinal Cleanse Program. You should also change your food choices to a low-fat, high-fiber diet that is mostly vegetarian, with only occasional fish or chicken. The gallbladder could release a larger stone that could block the bile duct, which would require immediate surgery.

If you determine The Gallbladder Flush is not for you right now, you can gently begin a gallbladder cleansing process with the following plan, including a nutritional-supplement formula that will facilitate the removal of fat from the liver and increase the solubility of the bile, and an herbal formula that will favorably affect the solubility of the bile. This program should dissolve any stones present and bring relief for gallbladder problems.

1. A lipotropic supplement, generally available at health food stores, includes choline, methionine, betaine, folic acid, and vitamin B_{12}. The herbal formula should include dandelion root, milk thistle, artichoke leaves, turmeric, and boldo.

2. Eat more fresh vegetables and fruits.

3. Take a gel-forming fiber such as psyllium husk or flaxseed daily.

4. Reduce your intake of saturated fats, cholesterol, sugar, and animal proteins. Completely avoid fried foods.

5. For one week, drink the following juices:

- *Carrot/beet/cucumber*. Drink three 8-ounce glasses per day.
- *Carrot/celery/endive*. Drink two 8-ounces glasses per day.

6. Drink the juice of one lemon with 8 ounces of hot water eight to ten times per day.

THE KIDNEY CLEANSE

The kidneys perform two important cleansing functions: They remove water and solutes, and they remove toxic waste from the blood. The typical Western pattern of eating low-fiber, highly refined carbohydrates; ingesting too much alcohol; eating large amounts of animal protein and fat; consuming high-calcium–containing foods, such as dairy products, which have less absorbable calcium than the calcium found in vegetables; and eating too much salt, contributes to kidney stones as well as weakened, less efficient kidneys.

Symptoms of possible kidney problems include blood in the urine, burning or pain during urination, cloudy urine, a cold sensation in the lower half of the body, dark circles under the eyes, frequent urination—especially at night, foul-smelling or dark urine, hypertension, incontinence, kidney stones, and pain in the eyes. Note: If you suspect kidney stones or have a urinary tract infection, see your doctor immediately.

The Kidney Cleanse Program

1. Drink plenty of purified water—8 to 10 glasses per day.

2. Daily drink 1 to 2 glasses of fresh juices that help to cleanse and support the kidneys. Choose from the following:

Asparagus/tomato/cucumber/lemon (Spring Tonic, page 33)

Cantaloupe, with seeds

Carrot/celery/parsley

Carrot/beet/coconut

Cucumber/mint

Watermelon

Stinging nettles/cucumber/lemon

*Cucumber, watermelon, cantaloupe, asparagus, lemon, kiwifruit, and
parsley juices* are good diuretics.

If you have a urinary tract infection, cranberry juice is recommended—see
Cran-Apple Cocktail, page 38.

3. Drink nettles tea. You can order Kidney Life Tea and Kidney Life herbal
supplements from Arise and Shine (800-688-2444).

THE LIVER CLEANSE

The liver is the largest internal organ of the body and one of the most
important. It performs a number of crucial functions: (1) metabolic functions, which involve carbohydrate, protein, and fat metabolism; (2) storage
of vitamins and minerals; (3) detoxification or excretion of chemical compounds such as hormones, drugs, and pesticides; (4) vascular functions, filtering over one liter of blood each minute and acting as a primary blood
reservoir; and (5) secretory functions, including synthesis and secretion of
bile; the liver manufactures about one liter of bile daily.

To a great extent your health and vitality depend on the healthy functioning of your liver. Optimizing liver function focuses on cleansing, protecting,
and nourishing the liver. A liver that is even slightly sluggish could quite
negatively affect your health. Exposure to toxic chemicals, drugs, alcohol, or
hepatitis, along with eating a typical Western diet, can create a sluggish liver.
It doesn't take megadoses of unhealthy substances to weaken the livers of
some people. For example, researchers have found that even small amounts
of alcohol can cause fat deposits in the livers of some individuals.

Symptoms of a sluggish liver include abdominal discomfort, aches and
pains, age spots (brown spots on the face and the backs of hands), allergies,
anal itching, bad breath, body odor, candidiasis, sallow or jaundiced complexion, coated tongue (whitish or yellow), constipation, digestive prob-

lems (belching, burping, and flatulence), dizziness, drowsiness after eating, fatigue, frequent urination at night (a weak liver can weaken the bladder and kidneys), headaches (feeling of fullness or heaviness in the head, with pain circling part of the head, the temples, or the eyes), hemorrhoids, inability to tolerate heat or cold, insomnia, irritability, loss of memory or inability to concentrate, loss of sexual desire, lower back pain, malaise, menstrual problems, migraine headaches, nervousness and anxiety, pain around the right shoulder blade and shoulder, PMS, puffy eyes and/or face, red nose, small red spots that look like moles (smooth or hard and raised), rheumatism, and sinus problems.

The 7-Day Liver Cleanse

Eat a vegan diet for seven days, which means excluding all animal products. Avoid alcohol, tobacco, sweets, and junk food completely. Add the following foods to your daily diet plan. If you miss a day, begin again.

Carrot Salad

Place 1 cup of finely shredded carrots or carrot pulp, left over from juicing, in a bowl. If shredding the carrots, they should be a mushy consistency; use a food processor or fine grater. (It's easiest to use carrot pulp.) Combine 1 tablespoon of extra-virgin, cold-pressed olive oil with 1 tablespoon of fresh lemon juice. You may add more olive oil and lemon juice, but not less. I like also to add a dash of cinnamon. Whisk the olive oil and lemon juice together in a small bowl. Pour the mixture over the shredded carrots or carrot pulp and mix well. Eat this salad every day for seven days.

Vegetable Broth

2 to 3 cups chopped fresh green beans
2 to 3 cups chopped zucchini
2 to 3 stalks chopped celery
1 to 3 tablespoons chopped parsley
1 tablespoon chopped garlic
Minced ginger, cayenne, vegetable seasoning, or herbs to taste

Steam green beans, zucchini, and celery over purified water until soft but still green. Put the vegetables in a blender and puree until smooth. Add a bit of the steaming water, if needed. The broth should be fairly thick. Season to taste. Eat one to two cups of the broth each day for seven days.

Fresh Beet Juice

Drink 3 to 8 ounces of fresh beet juice daily for seven days. Because of its strong taste, I recommend that you mix beet juice with other juices such as carrot, cucumber, endive, lemon, or apple. Beet juice has been used for decades to cleanse and support the liver. Endive has been used traditionally to promote the secretion of bile; this is helpful for the liver and gallbladder.

Milk Thistle (Silymarin)

Take one milk thistle capsule after each meal. Milk thistle contains some of the most potent liver-cleansing and protective compounds known. Silymarin, which is the active ingredient in milk thistle, enhances liver function and inhibits factors that cause hepatic damage. Because of its antioxidant properties, silymarin also helps prevents free-radical damage to the liver.

A product I have used and recommend is Liver Life by Arise and Shine. In addition to milk thistle, it contains artichoke leaf, dandelion root, bayberry root, bulpleurum, Oregon grape root, burdock root, black walnut hulls, wild yam root, fennel seed, stillingia root, and mandrake root. You can order this product by calling 800-688-2444.

Coffee Enema

Coffee enemas can help to remove toxins from the liver by causing the liver to produce more bile and stimulating bile flow. During this process, the liver can dump toxins into the bile quickly.

It is possible for a coffee enema to cause nausea because of the toxins that are being released. If this happens, drink several cups of herbal peppermint tea. This will help dilute the toxic bile overflow in the stomach and bring relief. (See page on enemas for more information.)

Note: Drinking coffee does not offer cleansing effects to the liver; it over-stimulates the adrenal glands and is not a healthful addition to your cleansing program.

1. *How to prepare the coffee enema:* Add 3 heaping tablespoons of ground, organically grown coffee* to one quart of purified water. Let it boil slowly for 3 minutes; then simmer for another 17 minutes with the lid on. Strain the grounds from the liquid and cool the liquid to body temperature.

2. *How to administer the coffee enema:* Lie down on your right side and draw both knees toward the abdomen. Take a deep breath before you release the contents of the enema bag to facilitate drawing the greatest amount of fluid into the colon. Retain the fluid for 12 to 15 minutes.

After the coffee enema, it is recommended that you drink an eight-ounce glass of carrot/celery juice since some minerals will be removed with the bile.

Take one or two coffee enemas over the course of The 7-Day Liver Cleanse.

Other beneficial juices that are good for the liver include apricot, chervil, dandelion, gooseberry, papaya, radish, string bean, tomato, and wheatgrass. There are numerous recipes that include these juices earlier in the book.

THE SKIN CLEANSE

The skin is the largest organ of the body. It has numerous functions, one of which is excretion. It assists the body in eliminating small amounts of water, salts, various organic compounds, toxins, and poisons. When other organs of elimination are overloaded, the skin will do everything possible to facilitate excretion. Since it acts as protection between the body and the millions of foreign substances in our environment, it can become overwhelmed and the body can react with pimples, bumps, acne, redness, rashes, scales, age spots, and other unsightly skin conditions.

---

*Note: Use only organically grown coffee because the chemicals used to grow conventional coffee are systemic (they have spread throughout the coffee beans) and would be counterproductive to the cleansing process of the coffee enema. They could add to the toxic load of the liver.

Whether your skin is dull, breaking out with pimples or bumps, showing signs of aging, or just needing more "life," a cleansing program will help it look healthier and more glowing. I recommend any of the cleansing programs in this section to improve your skin's health. Internal cleansing is very important because your skin reflects the inner state of your body. Beautiful, healthy skin begins on the inside. The following purge could help you with a jump start toward beautiful skin.

The Skin Purge Program

1. The following juices help to detoxify the skin. Drink at least two 8-ounce glasses of any of the following combinations per day for one week.

> *Cucumber/carrot/celery*
> *Cucumber/lemon* (Afternoon Refresher, page 18)
> *Apple/pineapple/cucumber* (Refreshing Complexion Cocktail, page 25)
> *Carrot/parsnip/green bell pepper* (Beautiful Skin, Hair, and Nails Cocktail, page 24)
> *Spinach/carrot* (Popeye's Power, page 21)
> *Asparagus/tomato* (Spring Tonic, page 33)

2. Drink eight to ten 8-ounce glasses of purified water per day during the cleanse and for the rest of your life.

3. Mt. Shasta Herb and Health has a skin cleansing program with three components: a mustard bath, herbal tea (to drink), and an herbal enema. You can order their Bring 'Em Back Alive Skin Purge by calling 888-343-7225.

ENEMAS AND COLONICS

Though not a practice to rely on daily, enemas are very helpful during all cleansing programs. The colon, kidneys, lungs, and skin can become overwhelmed with the release of toxins during a cleanse, and skin eruptions, headaches, and flu-type symptoms can result. Enemas assist the body in the elimination process and help minimize symptoms. Many people are not familiar with enemas today; however, their therapeutic benefits have been known for centuries. They were recorded as early as 1500 B.C. in an ancient Egyptian document. Hippocrates, the father of medicine, hailed their benefits. The Essenes, a monastic sect that flourished on the shores of the Dead

Sea at the time of Christ, wrote about their therapeutic function. After World War II, high-tech medicine dismissed this ancient healing practice, and consequently much of the Western population began to consider them unnecessary and undesirable. But enemas and colonics are making a comeback at the turn of the twenty-first century as a vital part of cleansing the body. (Colonics are high enemas that must be administered by a trained technician.)

BASIC GUIDELINES FOR THE VIBRANT HEALTH DIET

EAT A HIGH-FIBER, LOW-FAT, whole-foods diet. Complex carbohydrates (vegetables, whole grains, and legumes) should make up the largest portion of your food intake, with 15 to 20 percent from protein and 15 to 25 percent from fat. Although eating enough protein is important to overall health, there is evidence that too much protein can contribute to reduced immune function. Too much of the wrong types of fat (saturated and processed fats like margarine and hydrogenated oils) lower immune cell activity. The typical Western diet falls short on essential fatty acids (EFAs) found in cold-water fatty fish and unrefined seed and vegetable oils such as flaxseed, hemp, olive, and canola. EFAs are important to the healthy functioning of white blood cells.

Drink fresh juice; eat more raw foods. Raw food is *live food.* Make a large percentage of your carbohydrates raw fruits, vegetables, fresh juice, sprouts, seeds, and nuts if you want high-level health. What is "live food"? Once a fruit or vegetable is picked, it stops growing, but it is not "dead" in the sense of its energy field. The Kentons, authors of *Raw Energy* (Century Publishing, 1985) say that if we are "to penetrate the mysteries of raw energy, biochemists and nutritionists will need to acknowledge that the healing powers implicit in raw foods and their juices are greater than the sum of their parts as measured in terms of their nutrients and calories."

Don't you instinctively feel that eating green salads and fresh fruit and drinking freshly made juice is good for you? You may not know why you feel good about them, but the fact is they literally radiate energy, or what is termed *life force.* Plants contain a special form of energy directly derived from the sun during photosynthesis, and plants act as a transport system to get this light into our bodies. When we eat raw vegetables and fruits, this special energy is passed on to our cells. "Each cell of a raw apple, glass of carrot juice, or lettuce leaf, is oscillating [vibrating energy]," write Oldfield and Coghill in *The Dark Side of the Brain.* Electric currents are termed "alive," and therefore, all raw food, by reason of its electrical energy, is alive until the microcurrent is destroyed.

Researchers have found that cooking food destroys not just vitamins and enzymes, but the oscillating circuit within a plant's cells. Through a process known as *kirlian photography,* raw and cooked plants have been photographed to capture their energy rays. (Kirlian photography is a technique for making photographs of electrically conductive objects using no light source other than that produced by a luminous corona discharge at the surface of an object in a high-frequency electrical field.) I was amazed by the photographs taken by Harry Oldfield and reprinted in *The Dark Side of the Brain* (Element, 1991). Brilliant spikes of light, twinkling like stars, surrounded a raw cabbage head, while a cooked cabbage head revealed a dull, highly diminished corona discharge. Using the same techniques, Harry Oldfield photographed the hands of a person on a 24-hour, junk-food diet; the outline of the hands can barely be seen. Next he photographed the hands of a man who had eaten a whole-foods diet for 40 years; his hands showed energy rays and spikes completely surrounding them.

To move to a state of vibrant health and energy, nutritional experts recommend that you make 50 to 75 percent of your diet raw food: fruits, vegetables, juices, sprouts, seeds, and nuts. This high percentage may seem staggering until you consider that juicing can make up half of that percent, and it is fast and easy. Juicing enables you to quickly consume a lot of vegetables and fruits in a glass. Even if you do not reach the goal of 50 to 75 percent raw food, whatever steps you take in that direction are good.

Avoid fast food and pre-prepared foods. Most commercial foods are loaded with salt and/or sugar, preservatives, and additives. Too much salt causes sodium to be drawn into cells and potassium to be pulled out, and this imbalance leaves cells unable to absorb what they need or to excrete wastes and unwanted materials efficiently. Consequently, they cease to effectively carry out vital metabolic processes. Sugar will beat out vitamin C for absorption into white blood cells, thus impairing immune-system functions. Toxic wastes build up inside the cells and sludge accumulates outside. The symptoms of this clogging up and slowing down at the cellular level are fatigue, poor immune function, and ultimately disease.

SAMPLE VIBRANT HEALTH DIET MENU

Breakfast

Juice such as The Morning Energizer (page 16) or Morning Sunrise
(page 39) and toasted sprouted grain bread with nut butter or
muesli (see recipe in my cookbook, *The Healthy Gourmet*
[Clarkson Potter, 1996])

or smoothie with protein powder such as The Champ (page 56)
or Rise 'n' Shake (page 55)

Midmorning Energy Snack

Juice such as Parsley Pep (page 26) or The Ginger Hopper
(page 17) with vegetable sticks and/or $1/4$ cup raw nuts
or seeds

Lunch

Green leafy salad with tuna
and/or Cherie's Quick-Energy Soup (page 62)
and sprouted grain bread or whole-grain crackers

Midafternoon Energy Break

Juice such as Santa Fe Salsa Cocktail (page 19)
or Afternoon Refresher (page 18)
or smoothie such as Muscle Power Plus (page 56)
or Tropical Sunrise (page 55)

Dinner

Main course salad such as Chicken Curry Salad or Multi-Grain
Florentine Salad (recipes are from my cookbook *The Healthy
Gourmet*—main course salads incorporate lots of green leafy
vegetables with small amounts of animal protein or grains and
legumes)

and cup of soup or baked squash or sweet potato

or stir-fry with lots of vegetables and chicken, meat, seafood,
or tofu and brown rice

Evening Snack

Fresh fruit or juice such as Sweet Dreams Nightcap (page 29)
or herbal tea

DIET GUIDELINES

The following groups of foods make up the Vibrant Health Diet. For all categories, I recommend organically grown food. (For more information, see Organically Grown, page 180.) I have specified those foods that are recommended for this diet, as well as those foods that should be avoided.

Bread, Cereal, Rice, Pasta (6 to 11 servings per day)

For this group, a single serving is 2 slices of bread; $\frac{1}{2}$ cup dense cereal (hot or cold); 1 cup pasta; $\frac{3}{4}$ cup cooked rice.

Recommended Foods: All organically grown whole grains, such as rye, millet, buckwheat, whole wheat, cornmeal, oats, brown rice, wheat germ, bran. Whole grain pasta and noodles. Best bread choice: sprouted whole grain bread (baked at a very low temperature to preserve the life force; these breads can be found at most health food stores and must be refrigerated at all times). Snacks: air-popped popcorn, whole-grain crackers without added sugar or preservatives, baked whole-grain chips.

Foods to Avoid: White breads and crackers, refined flour pasta and noodles, refined and sugared cereals, potato chips, fried corn chips, fried potatoes, buttered/commercial popcorn, cakes, cookies, donuts, commercial muffins (high in sugar and fat).

Vegetables (a minimum of 3 to 5 servings per day)

For this group, a single serving is 1 cup lettuce or other leafy greens; $\frac{1}{2}$ cup cooked vegetables; 1 cup vegetable juice.

Recommended Foods: All organically grown fresh, raw, or lightly cooked vegetables. Steamed or baked potatoes (best choices are new red potatoes, sweet potatoes, yams); baked squash. All fresh vegetable juices.

Foods to Avoid: Canned vegetables. Fried vegetables. Canned or bottled vegetable juices, which are a secondary choice to fresh. Frozen vegetables are a secondary choice to fresh.

Fruits (2 to 4 servings per day)

For this group, a single serving is 1 medium whole fruit; $\frac{1}{2}$ cup chopped fruit; 1 cup fruit juice.

Recommended Foods: All fresh, raw, organically grown fruits and fruit juices.

Foods to Avoid: All canned fruits. Canned, bottled, or frozen juices, which are a secondary choice to fresh. Frozen fruit is a secondary choice to fresh.

Meat, Poultry, Fish, Beans, Eggs, and Nuts
(2 to 3 servings per day; 10 to 15 percent of daily calories)

For this group, a single serving is 4 ounces of cooked meat, poultry, or fish; $\frac{1}{2}$ cup dried beans or peas; 1 egg; 2 tablespoons nut butter; $\frac{1}{4}$ cup nuts or seeds.

Recommended Foods: Organically raised, skinless poultry and lean meat; all fish and seafood, but especially fatty cold-water fish such as salmon, tuna, mackerel, sardines, and trout for their omega-3 fatty acids. All beans, lentils, split peas, especially sprouted legumes such as bean and lentil sprouts. All soy products such as tofu, tempeh, and soy milk. All nuts, nut butters, seeds, and seed butters, especially sprouted seeds such as sunflower.

Foods to Avoid: Lunch or canned meats, hot dogs, bacon, sausage, organ meats (they store more toxins), fatty meats, charbroiled meats, fried chicken and red meat, poultry skin, all deep-fried products. Peanut butter with added oil and sugar. Nuts roasted in oil and/or salted. Refried beans with lard.

Milk, Yogurt, Cheese (2 to 3 servings, optional)

For this group, a single serving is 1 cup milk; 1 ounce of cheese; $\frac{1}{2}$ cup cottage cheese; 1 cup yogurt.

Recommended Foods: Organic dairy products. Choose low-fat milk, cheese, and plain yogurt. Growing numbers of people are allergic to or intolerant of dairy products. Dairy also tends to be quite mucus-forming. Calcium is plentiful in dairy products; however, you can also obtain calcium from dark leafy greens such as kale (very calcium-rich); corn tortillas with lime added; soy products; seeds, especially sunflower and sesame; and nuts, especially almonds. For milk, you can substitute fortified soy milk (especially good for women due to the protective activity of phytoestrogens), rice milk, or almond milk. You can substitute soy cheese for dairy cheese.

Foods to Avoid: Cheese with yellow dye (choose brands that are all natural); whole milk; sweetened yogurt; ice cream; sour cream.

Fats and Oils (recommended servings have not been determined; no more than 15 to 25 percent of your daily diet)

For this group, a single serving is 1 tablespoon butter or oil; 2 tablespoons salad dressing.

Americans eat too much saturated fat and not enough essential fatty acids (EFAs). Recommended oils rich in EFAs are as follows: Hemp oil contains a good balance of omega-3 and omega-6 fatty acids, as well as gamma-linolenic acid (GLA). Flaxseed oil is rich in omega-3 fatty acids. Soybean oil contains omega-3 and -6 fatty acids. A mixture of flaxseed oil and sesame or sunflower oil will offer a balance of omega-3 and omega-6 fatty acids. Extra-virgin olive oil is good, but contains smaller amounts of omega-3; it can be mixed with hemp or flaxseed oil, in equal parts, to improve the essential fatty acid balance. You can take 1 to 2 tablespoons per day of an essential fatty acid such as unrefined hemp or flaxseed oil as a supplement; mix hemp or flaxseed oil with juice or "chase" it with juice. You may also prepare dishes with any of the oils mentioned. Purchase only pure, unrefined, organic oils (they can be found at health food stores). For delicious recipes using flaxseed oil, get a copy of the book *Flax for Life* by Jade Butler. It can be found at health food stores or you can order it from Barlean's Organic Oils at 800-445-FLAX.

Some fish oils are associated with clean arteries and freedom from fatty degeneration. The health secrets of these oils revolve around two omega-3 fatty acids: eicosapentaenoic acid (EPA) and docosahexaenoic acid (DHA). Essential fatty acids in flaxseed, hemp, and several other oils provide the raw materials for our bodies to manufacture EPA and DHA. The richest sources of EPA and DHA are fatty cold-water fish such as salmon, herring, sardines, trout, and mackerel.

Avoid margarine, shortening, and partially hydrogenated oils—they contain trans-fatty acids; fried and deep-fried products and refined commercial oils contain toxic fatty acid derivatives. Trans-fatty acids and altered fatty acid derivatives can have adverse effects on cell membranes, brain development in infants, and on the cardiovascular, liver, and immune systems.

Miscellaneous

Recommended Foods: Herbal teas, green tea, garlic, ginger, herbal seasonings.

Foods to Avoid: Coffee, soft drinks, powdered drinks, alcohol, sweets, salt, anything with aspartame, preservatives, dyes, additives, or fake fat. All pesticide-sprayed produce and antibiotic-hormone-raised animals.

ORGANICALLY GROWN

WHY BUY ORGANICALLY GROWN? *Organic* refers not to the food itself, but to how it is produced. Organic foods are minimally processed to maintain the integrity of the food without artificial ingredients, preservatives, or irradiation. Organic food production is based on a system of farming that maintains and replenishes the fertility of the soil, and the plants are grown without the use of synthetic pesticides and fertilizers. Organic farmers are permitted to use natural botanical pesticides, which are derived from plants, as a last resort when crop failure is threatening. But their primary strategy is prevention. By building healthy soils, farmers grow healthier plants that are able to resist disease and insects.

It is not for better taste (although many chefs have found that organic food tastes better) or immediate health boosts that millions of people now reach for organically grown foods. Studies on pesticides and individual accounts of the detrimental effects these chemicals have on numbers of individuals are changing the minds of well-informed shoppers. Prevention, by omitting pesticides from our environment, may be our only salvation from agrichemically induced environmental illnesses.

Removing pesticides from his lifestyle was Steve's only hope. He went to see Dr. Walter Crinnion, N.D., after going to numerous doctors who had been unable to diagnose his problem; he thought he was dying. Dr. Crinnion found 9 of the 18 pesticides he was tested for in his blood. Steve went through an extensive protocol to remove the pesticides and eventually regained his health.

Steve is just one of the many thousands of people whose health has been adversely affected because of pesticides. The case of a 69-year-old woman was reported in the *Journal of Nutritional Medicine* (1991). Malnourished, weighing only 70 pounds, and diagnosed with amyotrophic lateral sclerosis and an inability to swallow, she was placed on total ventilatory support. This patient lived near a high-intensity, pesticide-spraying, chicken-raising operation. She had elevated levels of organochlorine pesticides and depressed T cells (immune cells). With prolonged ventilation and nutritional support, her T lymphocytes increased, pesticide levels decreased, and her health improved.

Over the past 30 years there has been a significant increase in the use of pesticide and nitrogen fertilizers for agricultural purposes—with both plants and animals. There are about 600 active pesticide ingredients. According to Dr. Dennis Weisenburger, M.D. (*Human Pathology*, 1993), human exposure to agrichemicals is common and can result in acute and chronic problems such as neurotoxicity, lung damage, chemical burns, infant methemoglobinemia, and some cancers.

Pesticides raise the risk of neurological problems, such as Alzheimer's and Parkinson's diseases, and developmental problems. They can also weaken the immune system, leaving us more vulnerable to disease. The Environmental Protection Agency (EPA) considers 60 percent of all herbicides, 90 percent of all fungicides, and 30 percent of all insecticides carcinogenic. Pesticides may cause an extra 1.4 million cancer cases among Americans, according to a 1987 National Academy of Sciences report.

Over the last three decades, our food supply has been fundamentally altered in the following ways:

- Chemical fertilizers are added to our soil. Pesticides and herbicides are sprayed on the crops, animals, and the ground. Chemicals are added to storage bins containing harvested food and animal feed.
- More petrochemicals are added to enhance taste and color of processed foods.
- The molecular structure of food is altered through irradiation.
- Biotechnology alters food at the genetic level.

There are many reasons to choose organic food. The most important is better health for ourselves and our loved ones. It is estimated that the average child today receives four times more exposure to widely used cancer-causing pesticides in food than has the average adult. "We have not inherited the Earth from our fathers, we are borrowing it from our children," says environmentalist Lester Brown. They are the best reason of all to choose organically grown foods.

Even if organically grown produce adds up to a few more cents at the cash register, it is saving us money in multiple ways. Organic farmers are preserving our air, soil, and water. Chemically dependent farming practices contribute to an annual erosion of 3 billion tons of topsoil. And then there are the directly related costs of agrichemical business. A recent Cornell University study added up the annual cumulative costs of chemical farming: $525 million damage to agricultural ecosystems, $250 million in pesticide-related illnesses and poisoning, $150 million for pesticide regulation and monitoring, and $1.3 million to test drinking water for pesticide contamination. If we think that organically grown is more expensive than chemically grown food, we need to look at the overall picture. The price of the chemicals is reflected not only in the price of our food, but in the cost of health care, the future of our soil, and the sustainability of our agricultural system.

WHAT ABOUT IRRADIATION?

There is an alarming new trend: the evolution of new and more lethal strains of bacteria that contaminate our food. At the time of this writing, the FDA has approved the use of nuclear radiation to decontaminate food. A report in the *Los Angeles Times* (December 1997) states that an average dose of radiation used to decontaminate most foods can be up to 5 million times as much as a typical chest X ray. This is a highly controversial practice because it destroys vitamins and minerals and generates dangerous by-products such as free radicals, released when gamma rays break up the molecular structure of the food. Free radicals can seriously damage cells (both membranes and DNA). (Free radicals are molecules that have lost an electron; they rob other molecules of electrons, damaging these molecules in a chain reaction.) Radiolytic products increased in irradiation include formaldehyde, benzene, formic acid, and quinones—all harmful to human health. One study found seven times as much benzene, a known carcinogen, in cooked irradiated beef than in cooked nonirradiated beef (*Food and Water Journal,* 1997). Irradiating fruits and vegetables poses an even greater problem because foods with high quantities of water are more vulnerable to the formation of free radicals.

Foodborne diseases in meats are caused in part by overcrowding on farms and in slaughterhouses, overuse of antibiotics (thus creating resistant strains of bacteria and viruses), unsanitary and unhealthy growing conditions for animals, and overuse of pesticides (sprayed on animals and their food). Irradiation is not the way to control the problem of foodborne bacteria in meats. The answer is to ensure more humane and sanitary growth conditions for the animals and more sanitary conditions at slaughterhouses and meatpacking plants. Similar recommendations apply for fruits and vegetables.

ARE ORGANICALLY GROWN FOODS MORE HEALTHFUL?

Organically grown foods usually have few, if any, chemical residues, and lower levels of nitrate nitrogen. A 1998 study (published in *Hort/Science*) indicated that organic food is more nutritious than inorganic, with organically grown tomatoes having more vitamin C and calcium than those cultivated inorganically.

CHOOSING ORGANICALLY GROWN

If you see food labeled "certified" organic, it has been grown according to strict uniform standards that are verified by independent state or private organizations. Certification includes inspections of farm fields and processing facilities, detailed record keeping, and periodic testing of soil and water to ensure that growers and handlers are meeting standards set by the government (1990) for produce, grains, meat, dairy, eggs, and processed food.

If food is labeled "transitional organic," it was grown in recently converted soil—or soil in the process of converting from chemical to organic.

WHAT IF ORGANIC ISN'T AVAILABLE?

If you can't find organic produce, add your voice to the chorus demanding that organically grown be available at your supermarket.

You also can search for small-operation farmers in your area. If you have a local farmers' market, talk to the purveyors displaying their produce about their farming practices. Many of them can't afford to use many chemicals in farming. Another option is to order organic produce by mail (see Appendix for names and addresses).

IV

CARROT JUICE FOR THE SOUL

It's not surprising to realize that many people became juicing converts after having an accident or being diagnosed with a serious physical ailment. Although each person's personal journey of healing is unique, they all have one thing in common—juicing on a daily basis not only helped heal them, but gave them vital life energy to feel and look better than they had in years.

THE MIRACLE CURE

Four years ago, 23-year-old Lisa Zentner was working as a ski instructor and golf pro in British Columbia. Despite being an avid outdoors-woman, Lisa didn't place much emphasis on the food she put into her body. Preparing balanced meals took too much time and energy—two vital things she would rather put into sports-related activities.

On the evening of May 22, 1994, Lisa gathered up her belongings after a long day's work and left the golf club where she was an instructor. She rode her bike over to her friend's house to wish her a happy birthday, but no one was home when Lisa arrived. She turned around and began her trip home, less than three miles away. As she coasted down a steep hill, the baseball cap she was wearing flew off her head. When she made a grab for her hat, she accidentally hit her front brake, causing her bike to stop short. She flipped over the handlebars and landed on her face, sliding several feet along the asphalt. As her belongings scattered all over the road, the only thing Lisa remembers saying to herself over and over again was, "I'm hurt, I'm really hurt." Bleeding profusely from her nose and lip, she somehow managed to get back on her bike and ride the rest of the way home. Her housemates put ice on her lip and nose in an attempt to stop the blood before taking her to the emergency room. Lisa still had no idea how bad the damage was to her face.

At the hospital, Lisa learned the extent of her injuries: her top lip was almost torn off, her nose broken, and her front teeth were bent up toward the roof of her mouth. Fourteen long needles had to be inserted into her lip to numb it before sewing it back up with an equal number of stitches. Along with the damage to her face, Lisa's entire body was battered and bruised. She was released from the hospital the same night as her accident, but put under the watch of her friends in case she lost consciousness. In the days that followed, Lisa had her nose set and her teeth splinted and moved back into place.

Unable to eat solid foods, the doctors suggested that she try ice cream, milk shakes, and yogurt. Lisa instinctively knew that loading up on dairy products and sugar could not provide her with the nutrients and energy she needed to heal. Wanda, her close friend and "guardian angel," borrowed a juicer from a coworker and gave it to Lisa, along with a copy of my book, *Juicing for Life*. Lisa began following juicing programs designed to help heal dental problems, skin abrasions, and rejuvenate the body after surgery. She wasn't thinking of juicing in terms of recovery, but as a way to get nourishment. Each day she had a large glass of pineapple juice, which promotes healthy gums, and a glass of carrot and broccoli juice to heal her torn skin. Startled by how fast her skin had begun to heal into healthy scabs, Lisa's doctor removed her stitches just four days after her accident. By the second week in June, just three weeks after her fall, Lisa's skin was completely healthy—the scabs had fallen off and there was virtually no scarring. Lisa's friends who had seen her at the time of the accident couldn't get over the speed of her recovery, and those who hadn't seen her had trouble believing that anything had ever happened.

By healing so quickly Lisa regained the sense of control she felt had been destroyed, which was just as vital to her emotionally and psychologically as her physical healing had been. Lisa attributes her speedy recovery, her much-improved endurance, and her uncanny new ability to ward off just about any strain of the cold or flu solely to juicing: "It's my miracle cure," she says.

A BANK ACCOUNT FOR THE FUTURE

Robyn Knapton Ridgly began juicing in her twenties while living in California. She had just graduated from college and wanted an easy way to get her daily vegetables. For her, juicing was the perfect answer. It was so simple, and it made her feel "alive." As she grew older and started her own business, Robyn began to have less and less time for juicing—and eating in general. Split between her family and her career, she began to feel run down. In her mid-thirties, she began to experience extreme bouts of fatigue accompanied by severe muscle pain. Within a year of first experiencing symptoms, Robyn was virtually bedridden—getting up to brush her teeth took all of her energy and willpower. Unable to continue a normal life, much less her career, Robyn was forced to give up her business.

Although Robyn was experiencing the onset of chronic fatigue syndrome, combined with anemia, it would be several years before doctors would be able to give her a definite diagnosis. Frustrated by seeing her life slip away in front of her eyes, Robyn decided she had nothing to lose by taking matters into her own hands. Relying on her good experiences with juice in the past, Robyn designed a vegetable and fruit juicing program that met the needs of her body, yet was simple and easy to prepare. She began drinking a combination of carrot, kale, and apple juice with every meal. Although it took several long months for her to regain her strength, drinking fresh juices each day provided Robyn with the energy she needed to get out of bed and rebuild her personal and professional life.

Now in her mid-forties, Robyn hasn't experienced fatigue symptoms in years, and her anemia has disappeared. She is a confirmed "juicer" and credits it as the driving force behind her vibrant health and youthful looks. When friends ask Robyn if it is difficult preparing fresh juices each morning, she tells them no, equating it to other daily routines such as taking a shower or brushing her teeth. "The key," she says, "is keeping it varied but *simple*." As the communications director for a congressman from Georgia, Robyn works long hours and is constantly on the go. Despite her daily stresses, she has learned to listen carefully to what her body is telling her. For example, if her body needs a late-afternoon lift, she'll drink a glass of apple, lemon, and ginger juice. It tastes surprisingly similar to lemonade and provides her with the zest she needs to finish out her day.

Robyn's husband Brad jumped on the juicing bandwagon two years ago when he was diagnosed with an acid reflux disorder. He began juicing whatever vegetable or fruit they had in the house, followed a low-fat diet, got moderate exercise, and eventually recovered completely from his illness. Robyn and Brad still start each morning with a nutrient-packed glass of carrots, sweet potatoes, kale, and beets. An inventor who frequently travels to Asia, Brad finds that juicing is also the perfect remedy for jet lag. He feels stronger now than he did in his twenties or thirties and resolutely believes that juicing is the most logical method of ensuring health and longevity. Along with the nutritional benefits, the ritual of juicing has afforded him the opportunity to explore his inner self and experience firsthand "the infinite intelligence and wisdom of the body."

YOU ARE WHAT YOU EAT

Gary Liss has been juicing for over two decades. He was first turned on to it as a method of healing upon his return from seven years of traveling through India, Asia, and Africa. When he got back to the States, he felt very weak. Gary, who had never had health problems before, went to his physician to see if she could help. He was diagnosed as suffering from a combination of "tropical diseases," including malaria and a strain of hepatitis that had done extensive damage to his liver. He was put on a cycle of antibiotics, but didn't place too much faith in their ability to repair his body. He knew that he needed to rebuild his immune system. After researching a number of alternative healing techniques, Gary came to the conclusion that food was the key. And it seemed logical that turning his vegetables into juice would be the quickest and easiest way to absorb their vitamins and minerals.

Gary immediately put himself on a strict body-maintenance program that included two glasses of fresh, organic carrot juice each day. He also changed his eating habits, consuming foods that were low in fat and high in protein in order to build muscle. After the first few days, he felt more alert and confident than he had in the past few years. As he grew more comfortable with juicing, he began to add spinach, beets, and other vegetables to his basic carrot juice.

Within the year, Gary had completely overcome his illnesses. His rapid recovery took everyone he knew, including himself, by surprise. What he learned about his body and its connection to food changed his life permanently. Even though he was still at an age where youth and vitality are taken for granted, he saw the unquestionable connection between food, body, and health.

Today, at age 47, Gary works out six days a week and feels that he is in the best shape of his life. A professional fitness trainer and bodybuilder who is often mistaken for being in his thirties, Gary has won one regional California bodybuilding competition and has appeared in several national fitness magazines, including *Iron Man* and *Men's Health and Fitness*. However, his real passion is helping people—particularly men and women in their late thirties and forties—begin their own journey of lifelong health. He designs fitness programs for his clients that increase their body consciousness through weight training, aerobics, and diet, always stressing that the *key* to health is staying natural. Gary wholeheartedly believes in the importance of including fresh, organic vegetable juices such as carrot, potato, spinach, and kale as essential components for revitalizing the body. To his clients he emphasizes that juicing is a simple way of getting the correct amount of daily nutrients into their systems and making themselves feel great.

FROM DEATH UNTO LIFE

In the summer of 1993, the last thing on John Cunningham's mind was cancer. A successful businessman and father of two, John was committed to living a healthy lifestyle that included a low-fat, no-meat diet combined with regular exercise. When he came down with a nagging cold, John didn't give it too much thought. After all, summer colds are a common, albeit annoying, part of the season. His cold turned into an earache, and after several weeks of taking antibiotics, his body still wasn't responding. By August, John was beginning to have a tightening feeling in his chest and started to have a difficult time breathing. He was taken to the emergency room, where doctors did several rounds of X rays and tests. At the age of 31, John was diagnosed with advanced-stage testicular cancer.

Having found 14 tumors in his body, including one the size of a football in his chest, John was immediately put on an aggressive cycle of chemotherapy. The tumor in his chest was growing at an alarming rate, and for three months John was subjected to lethal doses of radiation. His body was under siege from both the cancer and the radiation treatments. He developed a deadly blood disorder, TPT, as a direct result of his chemotherapy. The nerves in his legs were also destroyed, confining John to a wheelchair, and his spirits were rapidly fading due to constant pain and nausea.

John was released from the hospital for the final time the day before Thanksgiving. Both his family and his doctors knew he was dying. In a last-ditch effort to save his life, his physician suggested that if a donor could be found, a bone marrow transplant and surgery might give him more time. After three months of chemo treatments, John was so weak and unresponsive that he was unable to make his own medical decisions. Both his wife and father knew that he wouldn't survive another invasive treatment. His father had begun researching alternative therapies when John was first diagnosed. He decided that conventional medicine was not doing his son any good and instead sent him to the American Biologics Institute in Mexico—the place John credits for teaching him what he needed to know to save his life.

The philosophy behind American Biologics is reconnecting to your mind and body using natural healing techniques. When John arrived, his esophagus was torn from his continual vomiting. In the hospital, he had been fed intravenously. At the institute, John continued on a liquid diet, but this time he was fed a variety of organic vegetable and fruit juices. What the chemo could not do to save his life, juicing did. Within a short period of time,

John's tumors began to decrease in size. He regained the weight he had lost over the past months, increased his strength, and began to feel whole again. After leaving the institute, John continued following a juicing program.

In the first two years after his initial diagnosis, John drank two quarts of vegetable and fruit juice each day. He found that his body responded best to green vegetables and routinely drank a combination of cucumber, zucchini, and broccoli. He continued to maintain a low-fat, grain-and-vegetable-based diet. His doctors in Georgia were astounded by his progress but still unwilling to endorse his new, natural course of cancer treatment. They continued to pressure John to have surgery to remove the existing tumors even though they could clearly see they were decreasing in size on their own. John refused, knowing that surgery would only disrupt his healing process.

Today, five years later, half of John's tumors are gone, and the growth that was once the size of a football is benign and much smaller in size. Although John has cut down on the amounts of juices he drinks, he makes sure he has at least three 16-ounce glasses daily. He has learned to listen to what his body is telling him, and he chooses his juices accordingly, being careful to get a variety of greens into his body every day. And like most fathers, John is concerned about what his children are eating. Each afternoon he makes carrot and apple juice for himself and his two eldest children—he says it will probably be a while before his new baby develops a taste for such a concoction, but he's certain she will.

How Juicing Saved My Hair and Changed My Life!

Robert Farley (fictitious name) can be called an atypical, typical young man. Less than 10 years ago he ran his own successful business, went out with his friends on weekends, and basically thought very little about the connection between health and food. Because of his age and the fact that he "wasn't eating 10 pounds of meat a day," Robert considered himself relatively healthy. True, he was having recurring bouts of eczema, for which he took antibiotics, but he felt fine. His outlook changed considerably, however, when he noticed that his hair was starting to thin. He began to think that, despite what his doctors and pharmaceutical companies were telling him, his problem might not be strictly hereditary. Could his heavy meat and dairy–based diet be contributing to his hair loss? Could there be a nutritional answer to male pattern baldness?

After talking to a few vegetarian friends and reading several books on nutrition and health, Robert became aware of the disservice he was doing his body by eating animals. Not only was he adding unnecessary fat to his diet, he was unwittingly consuming growth hormones routinely fed to animals at large, factory-type farms. He began experimenting with different foods and found thousands of delightful, natural, unprocessed, pesticide-free alternatives. Because of his hectic lifestyle and frequent travel, he also needed to find ways to prepare meals without hassle. Then an acquaintance suggested that he buy a juicer, promising that it would be the best purchase of his life and do more for his physical health than any gym membership ever could.

Once Robert began drinking large glasses of carrot and cucumber juice every day, he noticed an incredible difference in his skin—his eczema eruptions occurred less frequently and with less and less severity. Eventually they disappeared entirely. His most exciting discovery, however, was something he hadn't even dreamed of: The carrot and cucumber juice seemed to be *reversing* his hair loss. He was incredulous at first, but the facts were right there, in the mirror. After regular consumption of carrot and cucumber juice for one year, his hair was beginning to grow back in a noticeable way. And not only was this solution completely natural and noninvasive, it cost significantly less than expensive medications and hair replacement treatments.

Robert also found juicing to be a pivotal factor in his recovery from minor surgery. Unable to eat comfortably, he drank a combination of spinach, carrot, and apple juice, which greatly reduced inflammation and gave him energy. Within five days, he was completely healed.

Being the type of person who gets to the roots of problems with practical solutions that don't merely mask symptoms, Robert found juicing was the ultimate way of eating, for three simple reasons: It was easy to find a diverse selection of fruits and vegetables at his local organic market; their nutrients were efficiently digested and used by the body; and perhaps most amazingly, his prep time for each glass was minimal. His faith in his new diet and juicing enabled Robert to achieve a heightened body consciousness and an increased awareness about meat consumption and its damaging effects to the environment. In addition, he had learned the importance of cutting through the blind faith we often give doctors and the medical establishment. What he found most absurd was the fact that doctors often prescribe medications that are toxic to the body and focus only on visible manifestations of an illness. The antibiotics he'd been given to treat his eczema often resulted in a chronic digestive disorder called "leaky gut syndrome." But Robert's belief in a more natural way of approaching healing led him to find an affordable, organic solution to a nagging problem by simply changing his diet. Today, he adamantly believes that if each of us would take as much time considering our health choices as we do our clothes, we'd all be living happier on a healthier planet.

HEART OF RECOVERY

When Bill Mayville, Sr., was diagnosed with heart disease at the age of 53, he was frightened. Bill had originally gone to the doctor for a regular exam, and had complained that he was often out of breath and generally felt tired and run down. His family doctor gave him a familiar prescription—aspirin, nitroglycerin pills, and most likely heart surgery. At the time of his diagnosis, Bill was under a tremendous amount of stress from his job. The added pressure of undergoing a potentially fatal surgery did not help matters. Bill had a hard time accepting his doctor's dire prognosis. He felt he was being coerced into a form of treatment that wasn't right for his body or his mind. His wife Patricia had been doing research into the world of natural healing prior to Bill's diagnosis and felt that Bill might find an answer to his health problems using an alternative therapy.

Both Bill and Patricia knew that by changing their diets and their relationship to food, they could become more attuned to the needs of their bodies. They decided to follow a strict vegan diet, eliminating all meat, dairy, and processed foods. Their diet revolved around juicing, the easiest and most efficient way to give their bodies the nutrients and benefits of raw vegetables. They also began taking vitamin supplements and herbs. Bill decided that his heart medications were toxic to his body, and told his physician that he would no longer be taking them—and to put the option of heart surgery on the back burner. He felt completely confident with his decision—he was giving his body what it was asking of him and instinctively knew it would work.

Bill and Patricia began drinking three 8-ounce glasses of juice with each meal. Because they could taste and feel a difference in their bodies when they juiced vegetables from large, commercial farms, they made a point of purchasing organically grown produce. Bill felt his body responded best to a combination of carrot, spinach or kale, and apple. Patricia would often add celery and parsley, along with beets every other day, to promote liver health. As with many people who juice on a regular basis, the couple felt a surge in their energy levels not long after beginning their program, and they noticed that they were less prone to minor ailments such as colds, headaches, and small aches and pains. But most important, Bill was healing his heart—within 18 months after his initial diagnosis, Bill had lost 45 pounds, no longer felt out of breath when walking or climbing stairs, and his stress levels were down. Although his physician remained skeptical, he admitted that Bill was well on his way to complete recovery.

Bill's illness and his recovery through a combination of body consciousness and diet have provided him and his wife with a much more optimistic outlook on their lives. By taking an active role in their health, they no longer have ambivalence—or fear—about what is going on in their bodies. This reassures them that they can handle the curves that life throws them. In addition, they now have the confidence to spread the word about the importance of establishing a lifelong connection to the body.

BRUNZI'S BEST

Like many people, Carol Marangoni derives great strength, friendship, and love from her animal companions. When her beloved golden retriever, Brunzi, was diagnosed with squamous cell carcinoma at the age of five, Carol was determined to do *anything* to save his life. She took Brunzi to see the chief oncologist at a prestigious New York veterinary hospital, confident that he would be able to help. She was told that Brunzi's only chance of survival would be to undergo immediate surgery to remove his cancerous lumps, followed by intensive chemotherapy treatments. Carol panicked. The thought of putting her friend through so much pain without any guarantees was devastating. When she asked about alternative therapies, the idea was quickly dismissed.

Carol knew there had to be a more humane answer and continued to explore her options. Her search led her to the office of Dr. Marty Goldstein, a holistic veterinarian, who counseled Carol to look beyond Brunzi's tumors and the idea of a quick cure, instead focusing on the underlying causes of the cancer. Brunzi's immune system was suppressed, and although this was due in part to genetics, his diet of commercial dog food, made with tremendous amounts of nutritionally deficient fillers and preservatives, was another large factor in his developing a deadly disease. Following Dr. Goldstein's advice, Carol began cooking Brunzi's meals herself, using fresh, organically grown vegetables, grains, and meats. She also baked preservative-free doggie treats, which were a big hit. This was supplemented with immune-boosting vitamins and minerals. Carol came up with the idea of juicing for Brunzi and her other dog Chaos all on her own. She was surprised at first that they would lap up every bit from their bowls. "I didn't think they would touch the juice, but it just made sense to give it a try. My dogs loved it!" Brunzi thrived on his new diet, and within a few months he was back to his old, playful self.

Brunzi lived five more healthy, happy years, but he eventually succumbed to a different form of cancer at the age of 10. Conventional veterinarians, however, were astounded that he had survived so long after his initial diagnosis. Carol continues to juice for Chaos, Mewey the cat, and the newest addition to her family, a seven-month-old puppy named Barnsberry. Much to her delight, they vie with each other to get first crack at the fresh juice of the day. Although they'll drink just about any vegetable juice she puts in front of them, she finds that they are particularly fond of a combination of carrot and spinach or carrot and kale juice. She'll often add an apple or pear to sweeten the concoction.

Brunzi's extraordinary success with juicing is just one of the many positive experiences Carol and her pets have had since they began their new diets. She notes that juicing keeps her friends' coats shiny and oil-free, their eyes bright, and their energy levels up. She said that she can especially notice the difference in her dogs' appearance when she compares them with animals she knows are being fed factory-produced foods. The latter, though energetic, lack the overall look of health and radiance that Chaos and Barnsberry have.

Carol's culinary reputation quickly spread among her neighborhood dogs and their caregivers. Demand for her treats and nutritional advice fired her entrepreneurial spirit. She gave up being a pharmacist and started Brunzi's Best, a mail-order catalog specializing in organic baked goods for dogs.

If you plan to introduce juicing into your pet's life, Carol suggests taking small, consistent steps—changing a dog's or cat's diet too rapidly can interfere with digestion. Remember that if they're used to processed foods, their bodies will continue to crave the artificial sweeteners that are routinely added. This might account for them turning up their noses at first to healthier fare. She recommends that you continue to feed your animal companion commercially produced food for the first few weeks. Add bits of vegetables to the food, slowly increasing the ratio of fresh food to canned or dried. You should also be giving them small bowls of fresh vegetable juice (avoid citrus fruits and tomatoes, as these are far too acidic for animals). Like many children, dogs and cats have a tendency to be finicky eaters, so you may have to test out several juice combinations before you find their favorite. As Carol says, "Don't give up, no matter how long it takes—your furry pals deserve the best!"

BRAIN FOOD FOR JASON

When Claire Phillips saw her grandson Jason (fictitious names) right after his birth, he seemed to be a healthy baby despite being born to parents who abused alcohol and drugs. Due to her daughter's addiction, Claire's relationship with her was strained at best. Although they spoke periodically on the phone, Claire did not see Jason again until he was two years old. When he finally came for a visit, she could immediately see that Jason was being neglected by his parents. He was very thin and anxious from being left alone for long periods of time. His diet consisted of heavily processed foods, with little or no fresh fruits or vegetables. Jason's skin was raw and sensitive to the touch, he had acute allergies, intestinal problems, recurring temper tantrums, and fits of acting out. His mother admitted that he had been suffering from constant colds and infections and was regularly on antibiotics, though they seemed to be having little, if any, benefit. Claire knew her daughter was still abusing drugs and therefore incapable of caring for Jason. As emotionally draining and difficult as it was to take a baby from his mother, Claire felt it was the only way she could save him. After coming to an agreement with her daughter, she and her husband took Jason into their home.

Having raised several children, Claire knew the types of foods children need to grow healthy and strong. She also knew that Jason needed stability and routine. Claire established a regular eating schedule and tried to make sure that he got plenty of rest. As Jason grew older, it became apparent that he was having difficulty concentrating—he couldn't sit still for any period of time and would become easily frustrated. Suspecting that Jason might have attention deficit disorder (ADD), she began attending workshops and seminars on ADD and fetal alcohol syndrome. A British physician specializing in ADD told her that most children who suffer from these disorders didn't get enough nutrients in the womb. As a result, they have trouble filtering out the barrage of stimuli they receive from the world around them. After seeing several doctors, Jason was officially diagnosed with ADD. Claire knew, however, that medicating him was not the answer. She was interested in treating the causes of Jason's emotional and physical problems, not their manifestations. She felt that his poor diet as an infant was most likely the largest contributing factor to his hyperactivity and susceptibility to colds and other childhood illnesses. She also realized that changing his diet would be the simplest and most healthy type of treatment for Jason.

Claire found that putting a young child on a whole-foods diet wasn't as difficult as she'd thought, but it did require a little ingenuity and creativity on her part. She began by phasing out all packaged and refined foods, sugar, and food colorings. She immediately saw the difference in Jason. So did his counselor and teacher. When he didn't eat sugar, he was much calmer, could focus on games and tasks better, and didn't act aggressively toward other children. Claire turned eating fruits into fun by making "shakes" (that's how she got her own children to eat healthy foods 20 years previously) by mixing bananas, strawberries, pears, and any other fruits she had in the house together with a little milk or fresh orange juice. She was careful to avoid giving him apples—their natural silicates tended to make him more excitable.

As Jason became used to eating fresh foods, Claire introduced vegetable combinations such as carrot with pineapple and grapefruit, or spinach and kale with pineapple. She found that the easiest way to get him excited about eating healthfully was to turn it into a game. Instead of drinking carrot and spinach juice, Jason was having a "power drink" (the same drink that all his favorite superheroes had before bedtime)—bean sprouts became "ninja sprouts" (these have turned out to be one of Jason's all-time favorite snack foods), and favorite fruit juices were "brain food." After speaking with her physician, she added supplements to his diet, including a chewable form of acidophilus, which replaces intestinal flora and aids digestion, and *efmol focus,* a combination of evening primrose oil, tuna oil, and vitamin E, which acts as a natural stress reliever.

Claire is continually amazed by the turnaround in Jason's behavior, and she confidently attributes it to his diet and a loving family atmosphere. She describes Jason as being very "alive and inquisitive." Unlike the nervous child she first met four years ago, Jason is energetic, outspoken, and always exploring the world around him. He plays on his local soccer and baseball teams, and he just graduated from his third-level swimming class. She also finds that he is incredibly mature for a boy his age. He realizes that he's "different" from other kids but wants to be able to fit in and play with them. He seems to know that it's because of his healthy diet that he no longer acts "wild." He doesn't put up much of a fuss over what he gets to eat, though Claire has to hide his weekly potatoes in his spinach juice. In fact, he's so accustomed to eating right that on the rare occasions when Claire forgets to give him his vitamins, he'll go over to the cabinet and get them out himself, but not before shaking his finger and scolding her! "Juicing," Claire says, "has been the easiest way for me to get nutrients into Jason. Children are finicky eaters and often have sensitive stomachs. By giving Jason vegetables and fruits in their purest form, I know he's getting almost everything he needs to grow."

THE BREATH OF LIFE

Ten years ago, Mary Lou Arrington thought she was dying. When she first began experiencing symptoms that included constant fatigue, joint pain, and debilitating backaches, her doctors diagnosed her with early menopause and told her that, in time, her body would adjust. However, Mary Lou continued to grow worse. Her pain and exhaustion increased until she reached the point where even eating was a trial for her. She also began to get lumps on her back. By the time she went to see her doctor again to have her condition reevaluated, her back was bent at a dramatic angle. Her doctor ran a battery of tests on her, told her that the lumps were nothing more than fibrous tissue, and then returned with a devastating diagnosis: cancer. He told Mary Lou's husband that she had 30 days to live. Unbeknownst to Mary Lou, her family, and her doctors, she was suffering from tuberculosis (TB). Her doctors had never bothered to test her for TB, even though she told them that she had spent two years teaching English in Osaka, Japan, and had traveled extensively through China. Much to the embarrassment of Mary Lou's doctors, a nurse who worked in the hospital recognized her symptoms and ran a simple blood test, confirming her preliminary suspicions of TB.

The disease settled in her lungs and ovaries. Mary Lou's back problem was a result of Pott's disease, an illness marked by a curvature of the spine and most often associated with TB. She was immediately hospitalized and began a course of treatment that included taking extensive amounts of medications. When she was released, Mary Lou was literally starving, while still experiencing tremendous bouts of pain that left her bedridden. Unable to eat, she had deprived her body of the vitamins and minerals it needed to recover and mend. Her mother came to take care of her, preparing large plates of fresh vegetables each day. However, chewing took all of Mary Lou's energy, and after several days of trying to eat, she was exhausted. Then she saw a juicing infomercial on TV and knew that this was her ticket to a healthy life.

She began juicing six or seven 8-ounce glasses of juice a day. She combined a variety of fruits and vegetables together, including beets, carrots, fresh ginger, kale, spinach, apples, strawberries, blackberries, and grapefruit. In each glass, she mixed in mineral and protein powder supplements purchased from her local health food store. After one month, she experienced a difference in her body and mind. Her pain was all but gone, which lifted her spirits tremendously and gave her the will to fight back and heal. Then the lumps on her back disappeared. Finally she was able to stand upright once again. When she went back to her primary doctor after six months of juicing, her physical recovery was so dramatic that he didn't recognize her as she sat in his waiting room.

Mary Lou believes that when she became extremely ill, she hit a wall—a wall constructed by a medical system designed to treat masses of people instead of individual needs. By taking control of her illness and using a natural, organic treatment, Mary Lou discovered an entirely different approach to well-being, one that strives to uncover and heal the roots of disease instead of focusing on treating its symptoms. The true rewards of this life journey, she learned, come from an understanding of the relationship between food and the body. This new knowledge gave her the fortitude to stand up to conventional doctors who were continuing to pressure her to undergo expensive treatments, including a preventive pulminectomy (lung removal), despite her extraordinary recovery through juicing. Her courage saved her life, and her lung, and enabled Mary Lou to connect with an entire community of people whose heightened consciousness benefits not only their own well-being, but that of the planet as well.

Mary Lou has not experienced any pain or symptoms of TB for several years. She continues to juice vegetables, wheatgrass, and fruits every day, maintaining that it is the most important element of her overall health program. She uses herbs such as echinacea, vitamin C, and cayenne pepper to boost her immune system, follows a low-fat diet, and swims daily. Mary Lou feels better than she has in her entire life, and she attributes every ounce of her newfound energy to better nutrition through juicing and eating right.

Appendix

Information and Supplies

HEALTH INSTITUTES THAT OFFER JUICE PROGRAMS

Hippocrates Health Institute
1443 Palmdale Court
West Palm Beach, FL 33411
800-842-2125

Optimum Health Institute of Austin
Route 1 Box 339J
Cedar Creek, TX 78612
512-303-4817

Optimum Health Institute of
San Diego
6970 Central Ave.
Lemon Grove, CA 91945-2198
619-464-3346 or 800-993-4325

ORGANICS

Organic Produce by Mail

Walnut Acres Organic Farms
Penn Creek, PA 17862
800-433-3998

Diamond Organics
P.O. Box 2159
Freedom, CA 95019
800-922-2396

Information on Organic Production

Campaign for Sustainable Agriculture
12 N. Church Street
Goshen, NY 10924
914-294-0633

Environmental Working Group
1718 Connecticut Avenue, NW
Suite 600
Washington, DC 20009
202-667-6982

Mothers and Others for a Livable Planet
40 West 20th Street
New York, NY 10011
212-242-0010

The Organic Food Alliance
2111 Wilson Boulevard,
Suite 531
Arlington, VA 22201
703-276-9498

Organic Foods Production of North
America
P.O. Box 1078
Greenfield, MA 01302

Mail Order Organic Doggie Treats—
"Doggie Divines"
Brunzi's Best
RR1 Box 63
Garrison, NY 10524
914-734-4490
Fax: 914-737-7415

"Love of Animals" Newsletter
Natural Care and Healing for Your Pets
Dr. Bob and Susan Goldstein
800-711-2292

Earth Animal Outreach
Susan Goldstein, Pet Nutritionist
800-622-0260

Northern Skies Veterinary Center
(202) 222-0260
Bob Goldstein, V.M.D.
Wholistic Veterinary Services

Blood analysis/immune system test matches animal's blood with optimal immune system program. The test detects imbalances in an animal's immune system and enables Dr. Goldstein to customize a healing program for the animal.

Bibliography

Why Juice?

Batmanghelidj, By F., M.D. *Your Body's Many Cries for Water.* Falls Church, VA: Global Health Solutions, Inc., 1995.

Murray, M. T. *Encyclopedia of Nutritional Supplements.* Rocklin, CA: Prima Publishing, 1996.

Schardt, David. "Phytochemicals: Plants Against Cancer," *Nutrition Action Newsletter,* April 1994; 21(3):7–13.

Skerrett, P. J. "Mighty Vitamins: The One-A-Day Wonders Bidding to Outstrip Their Role as Supplements," *Medical World News,* January 1993; 24–32.

Wang, Hong, et al. "Total Antioxidant Capacity of Fruits," *Journal of Agricultural and Food Chemistry,* 1996; 44:701–705.

"What's the Best Diet?" *Nutrition Action Health Letter,* December 1991; 71:7–9.

Yamahara, J., et al., "The Anti-Ulcer Effect in Rats of Ginger Constituents," *Journal of Ethnopharmacology,* 23:299–304.

Vegetable-Fruit Juice Combinations

Albert-Pudeo, M. "Physiological Effects of Cabbage with Reference to Its Potential as a Dietary Cancer-Inhibitor and Its Use in Ancient Medicine," *Journal of Ethnopharmacology,* December 1983; 9(2):261–272.

Barale, R., et al. "Vegetables Inhibit, in Vivo, the Mutagenicity of Nitrite Combined with Nitrosamine Compounds," *Mutation Research,* 1983; 120:145–150.

Block, G. "Dietary Guidelines and the Results of Food Consumption Surveys," *American Journal of Clinical Nutrition,* 1991; 53:356S–357S.

Canty, D. J. and Zeisel, S. H. "Lecithin and Choline in Human Health and Disease," *Nutrition Reviews,* 1994; 52:327–339.

Cheney, Garnet, et al. "Anti-Peptic Ulcer Dietary Factor (Vitamin 'U') in the Treatment of Peptic Ulcer," *Journal of the American Dietetic Association,* 1950; 26:688–672.

Gerster, Helga. "The Potential Role of Lycopene for Human Health," *Journal of the American College of Nutrition,* 1997; 16(2):109–126.

Lassus, A. "Colloidal Silicic Acid for Oral and Topical Treatment of Aged Skin, Fragile Hair, and Brittle Nails in Females," *Journal of International Medical Research,* 1993; 21:209–215.

Ramon, Jose M. "Dietary Factors and Gastric Cancer Risk: A Case-Controlled Study in Spain," *Cancer,* March 1, 1993; 71(5):1731–1735.

Sable-Amplis, R., et al. "Further Studies on the Cholesterol-Lowering Effect of Apple in Humans: Biochemical Mechanisms Involved," *Nutrition Research,* 1983; 3:325–328.

Srivastava, K. C. and Mustafa, T. "Ginger (*Zingiber Officinale*) in Rheumatism and Musculoskeletal Disorders," *Medical Hypothesis,* 1992; 39:342–348.

Tsai, Y., et al. "Antiviral Properties of Garlic: In Vitro Effects on Influenza B Herpes Simplex and Coxsackie Viruses," *Planta Medica,* October 1985; 5:460–461.

Fruit Juice Recipes

Altman, R., et al. "Identification of Platelet Inhibitor Present in the Melon (*Cucurbitacea Cucumis Melo*)," *Thrombosis and Haemostatis,* 1985; 53(3):312–313.

Blau, L. W. "Cherry Diet Control for Gout and Arthritis," *Texas Reports on Biology and Medicine,* 1950; 8:309–311.

Bone, M. E., et al. "Ginger Root—A New Antiemetic," *Anesthesia,* 1990; 45:669–671.

Konowalchuk, J., et al. "Antiviral Effects of Apple Beverages," *Applied and Environmental Microbiology,* December, 1978; 36(6):798–801.

Lagrue, E., Behar, A., Maurel, P. "Edematous Syndromes Caused by Capillary Hyperpermeability," *Journal des Maladies Vasculaires,* 1989; 14:231–235.

Mann, Denise. "Purple Grape Juice, Wine and Beer All Cardioprotective," *Medical Tribune,* May 1, 1997; 26.

Mubagwa, K., et al. "Role of Adenosine in the Heart and Circulation," *Cardiovascular Research,* 1996; 32:797–813.

Rao, C., Rao, V., and Steinman, B. "Influence of Bioflavonoids on the Metabolism and Crosslinking of Collagen," *Italian Journal of Biochemistry,* 1981; 30:259–270.

Skerrett, P. J. "Mighty Vitamins: The One-A-Day Wonders Bidding to Outstrip Their Role as Supplements," *Medical World News,* January 1993; 24–32.

Sobota, A. E. "Inhibition of Bacterial Adherence by Cranberry Juice: Potential Use for the Treatment of Urinary Tract Infections," *Journal of Urology,* 1984; 131:1013–1016.

Srivastava, K. C. and Mustafa, T. "Ginger (*Zingiber Officinale*) in Rheumatism and Musculoskeletal Disorders," *Medical Hypothesis,* 1992; 39:342–348.

Tassman G., Zafran, J., and Zayon, G. "Evaluation of a Plant Proteolytic Enzyme for the Control of Inflammation and Pain," *Journal of Dental Medicine,* 1964; 19:73–77.

Fizzes

Bykowski, Mike. "Unhealthy Liquids May Promote Obesity," *Family Practice News,* March 1, 1997; 61.

"Obesity, Growth and Fruit Juice," *Pediatrics,* January 1997; 99(1):15–22.

Smoothies

Clausen, S. W. "Carotenes and Resistance to Infection," *Transactions of the American Pediatric Society,* 1931; 43:27–30.

Colquhoun, David M., et al. "Comparison of the Effects on Lipoproteins and Apolipoproteins of a Diet High in Monounsaturated Fatty Acids, Enriched with Avocado and a High Carbohydrate Diet," *American Journal of Clinical Nutrition,* 1992; 56:671–677.

Keen, C. L., and Zidenberg-Cherr, S. "Manganese," *Present Knowledge in Nutrition, 6th Edition,* Brown, M. L. (ed.), International Life Sciences Institute, Washington, D.C., 1990; 279–286.

Mann, Denise. "Strawberries, Spinach as Powerful as Vitamins in Antioxidant Activity," *Medical Tribune,* September 18, 1997; 3L.

Whitteman, J. C. M., et al. "Reduction of Blood Pressure with Oral Magnesium Supplementation in Women with Mild to Moderate Hypertension," *American Journal of Clinical Nutrition,* 1994; 60:129–135.

Look Younger

"Aging," *Nutrition Week,* May 17, 1996; 6.

Berger, K. *The Developing Person Through the Life Span.* New York: Worth Publishers, 1983, 519–531.

Cheraskin, E. "Chronologic versus Biologic Age," *Journal of Advancement in Medicine,* spring 1994; 7(1):31–41.

Cutler, R. "Carotenoids and Retinol: Their Possible Importance in Determining Longevity of Primate Species," *Proceedings of the National Academy of Sciences of the United States of America,* 1984; 81:7627–7631.

Leibovitz, B., and Siegel, B. "Aspects of Free Radical Reactions in Biological Systems: Aging," *Journal of Gerontology,* 1980; 35:45–60.

McDonald, R. "Influence of Dietary Sucrose and Biological Aging," *American Journal of Clinical Nutrition,* 1995; 62(suppl.):284S–293S.

Meydani, M., et al. "Vitamin E Requirements in Relation to Dietary Fish Oil and Oxidative Stress in Elderly," *Free Radicals and Aging,* 1992; 411–418.

Murray, M. *Encyclopedia of Nutritional Supplements.* Rocklin, CA: Prima Publishing, 1996.

Olivieri, O. "Selenium Status, Fatty Acids, Vitamins A and E and Aging: The Nove Study," *American Journal of Clinical Nutrition,* 1994; 60:510–517.

Poeggeler, B., et al. "Melatonin, Hydroxyl Radical-Mediated Oxidative Damage, and Aging," *Journal of Pineal Research,* 1993; 14:151–168.

Ward, J. "Free Radicals, Antioxidants and Preventative Geriatrics," *Australian Family Physician,* July 1994; 23(7):1297–1305.

Weindruch, R. "Calorie Restriction and Aging," *Scientific American,* January 1996; 46–52.

Prevent or Correct Age Spots

Balch, J. F., Balch, P. A. *Prescriptions for Nutritional Healing.* Garden City Park, NY: Avery Publishing Group, Inc., 1993.

Bolognia, J. L. "Aging Skin," *American Journal of Medicine,* January 1995; 98:99S–103S.

Bolognia, J. L. "Dermatological and Cosmetic Concerns of Older Women," *Clinics in Geriatric Medicine,* February 1993; 9:209–229.

Buchman, D. D. *The Complete Herbal Guide to Natural Health and Beauty.* New Canaan, CT: Keats Publishing, Inc., 1995.

Darr, D., et al. "Effectiveness of Antioxidants (Vitamin C and E) With and Without Sunscreens as Topical Photoreceptors," *Acta Dermato-Venereologica,* July 1996; 74:264–268.

Editors of Time-Life Books, *The Medical Advisor.* Alexandria, VA: Time Life Books, 1996.

Ford, N. *18 Ways to Look and Feel Half Your Age.* New Canaan, CT: Keats Publishing, Inc., 1996.

Holxle, E. "Pigmented Lesions as a Sign of Photodamage," *British Journal of Dermatology,* September 1992; 127:48–50.

Kanter, M. M. "Free Radicals, Exercise, and Antioxidant Supplementation," *International Journal of Sports Nutrition,* 1994; 4:205–20.

Keegan, L. *Healing Nutrition.* Albany, NY: Delmar Publications, 1996.

Lust, J. B. *Raw Juice Therapy.* London: Thorsons Publishers Limited, 1971.

Ponce, M. "The Formation of Competent Barrier Lipids in Reconstructed Human Epidermis Requires the Presence of Vitamin C," *Journal of Investigative Dermatology,* September 1997; 109:348–355.

Pritchard, P. *Healing with Whole Foods.* Berkeley, CA: North Atlantic Books, 1993.

Simon-Schnass, I. M. "Nutrition and High Altitude," *Journal of Nutrition,* 1992; 122:778–781.

"Skin Savers: Shade Your Skin from the Inside," *Prevention,* February 1994; 46:12.

Tant, L. "The Latest Way to Take Your Vitamins," *Chatelaine,* February 1998; 71:62.

Wallach, J. D. *Rare Earth's Forbidden Cures.* Bonita, CA: Double Happiness Publishing Co., 1996.

Yu, B. P. *Free Radicals in Aging.* Boca Raton, FL: CRC Press, 1993.

Prevent or Correct Cellulite

Draelos, Z. D., Marenus, K. D. "Cellulite: Etiology and Purported Treatment," *Dermatologic Surgery,* 1997; 23:1177–1181.

Gardner-Abbate, S. "New Insight on the Etiology and Treatment of Cellulite According to Chinese Medicine: More than Skin Deep," *American Journal of Acupuncture,* 1995; 23:339–346.

Lotti, T., et al. "Proteoglycans in So-Called Cellulite," *Journal of Dermatologic Surgery and Oncology,* 1990; 29:272–274.

Murray, M., Pizzorono, J. "Cellulite," *Encyclopedia of Natural Medicine,* 2nd ed. Rocklin, CA: Prima Publishing, 1998.

Nurnberger, F., Muller, G. "So-Called Cellulite: An Invented Disease," *Journal of Dermatologic Surgery and Oncology,* 1978; 4:221–229.

Scherwitz, C., Braun-Falco, O. "So-Called Cellulite," *Journal of Dermatolic Surgery and Oncology,* 1978; 4:230–234.

Van Straten, M. *Healing Foods: Nutrition for the Mind, Body, and Spirit,* Greenfield, M., ed. New York: Barnes & Noble, 1997.

Wormwood, V. A. *The Complete Book of Essential Oils & Aromatherapy.* San Rafael, CA: New World Library, 1991.

Healthy Hair and Nails

Balch, J. F., and Balch, P. A. *Prescriptions for Nutritional Healing.* Garden City Park, NY: Avery Publishing Group, Inc., 1990.

Buchman, D. *The Complete Guide to Natural Health and Beauty.* New Canaan, CT: Keats Publishing, 1973.

Eller, M. S. "Epidermal Differentiation Enhances CRABP II Expression in Human Skin," *The Journal of Investigative Dermatology,* December 1994; 103:785–789.

Finzi, E. "Cellular Localization of Retinoic Acid Receptor-Gama Expression in Normal and Neoplastic Skin," *American Journal of Pathology,* June 1992; 6(1):1463–1470.

Keegan, L. *Healing Nutrition.* Albany, NY: Delmar Publishers, 1996.

Lust, J. B. *Raw Juice Therapy.* London: Thorsons Publishers Ltd., 1958.

Olivares, M. "Copper as an Essential Nutrient," *American Journal of Clinical Nutrition,* May 1996; 63:791S.

Pitchford, P. *Healing with Whole Foods.* Berkeley, CA: North Atlantic Books, 1993.

Sato, S. "Iron Deficiency: Structural and Microchemical Changes in Hair, Nails, and Skin," *Seminars in Dermatology,* December 1991; 10:313–319.

Smith, L. *Feed Yourself Right.* New York: McGraw-Hill Book Co., 1993.

Stumpf, W. E. "Distribution of 1,25-dihydroxyvitamin D3922-oxal in Vivo Binding in Adult and Developing Skin," *Archives of Dermatological Research,* 1995; 87:294–303.

Wallach, J. D. *Rare Earths Forbidden Cures.* Bonita, CA: Double Happiness Publishing Co., 1994.

Williams, D. "Transectional Level Dictates the Pattern of Hair Follicle Sheath Growth in Vitro," *Developmental Biology,* 1994; 165:469–479.

Healthy Skin

Balch, J. F., Balch, P. A. *Prescriptions for Nutritional Healing.* Garden City Park, NY: Avery Publishing Group, Inc., 1990.

Boxer, A., Back, P. *The Herb Book.* London: Hamlyn, 1992.

Buchman, D. D. *The Complete Guide to Natural Health and Beauty.* New Canaan, CT: Keats Publishing, Inc., 1973.

Djerassi, D. "The Role of the Corrective Vitamins A, B_5, and C in the New, High Performance Cosmetics," *Drug and Cosmetic Industry,* June 1997; 160:60–63.

Erasmus, U. *Fats That Heal; Fats That Kill.* Burnaby, BC: Alive Books, 1993.

Gursche, S. *Healing with Herbal Juices.* Burnaby, BC: Alive Books, 1993.

Heinerman, J. *Heinerman's Encyclopedia of Healing Juices.* Englewood Cliffs, NJ: Prentice Hall, 1994.

Kenton, L., Kenton, S. *Raw Energy.* London: Century Publishing, 1985.

Lust, J. B. *Raw Juice Therapy.* London: Thorsons Publishers Limited, 1958.

Murray, M. T. *The Encyclopedia of Nutritional Supplements.* Rocklin, CA: Prima Publishing, 1996.

"Perfect Skin (Almost): Fast Fixes for the Top 6 Problems—From Fine Lines to Age Spots," *Good Housekeeping,* September 1996; 223:44.

"Skin Savers: Shade Your Hide from the Inside," *Prevention,* February 1994; 46:12.

Swain, R. "Vitamins as Therapy in the 1990s," *Journal of American Board of Family Practice,* May/June 1995; 8:206.

High-Level Energy

Benton, D., Cook, R. "The Impact of Selenium Supplementation on Mood," *Biological Psychiatry,* June 1991; 29(11):1092–1098.

Ellis, F. R., Nasser S. "A Pilot Study of Vitamin B_{12} in the Treatment of Tiredness," *British Journal of Nutrition,* 1973; 30:277–283.

Haas, E. M. *Staying Healthy with Nutrition.* Berkeley, CA: Celestial Arts, 1992.

Hoffman, D. *The Herbal Handbook: A User's Guide to Medical Herbalism.* Rochester, NY: Healing Arts Press, 1988.

Kenton L., Kenton S. *Raw Energy.* London: Century Publishing, 1985.

Murray, M., Pizzorno, J. *Encyclopedia of Natural Medicine.* Rocklin, CA: Prima Publishing, 1991.

Oldfield, H., Coghill, R. *The Dark Side of the Brain.* Rockport, MA: Element, Inc., 1991.

Pedersen, M. *Nutritional Herbology,* 2nd ed. Warsaw, IN: Wendell W. Whitman Co., 1994, 28.

Pitchford, P. *Healing with Whole Foods.* Berkeley, CA: North Atlantic Books, 1993.

Pizzorno, J. E., Murray, M. T. *The Textbook of Natural Medicine.* Seattle, WA: Bastyr University Publications, 1992.

Longevity

Cheraskin, E. "Chronologic Versus Biologic Age," *Journal of Advancement in Medicine,* Spring, 1994; 7(1):31–41.

Cutler, R. "Carotenoids and Retinol: Their Possible Importance in Determining Longevity of Primate Species," *Proceedings of the National Academy of Sciences of the United States of America,* 1984; 81:7627–7631.

Kenton, L., Kenton, S. *Raw Energy.* London: Century Publishing, 1985.

Lai, Chai-Nan. "Chlorophyll: The Active Factor in Wheat Sprout Extract Inhibiting the Metabolic Activation of Carcinogens in Vitro," *Nutrition and Cancer,* 1978; 1:3.

Leibovitz, B., Siegel, B. "Aspects of Free Radical Reactions in Biological Systems: Aging," *Journal of Gerontology,* 1980; 35: 45–60.

Meydani, M., et al. "Vitamin E Requirements in Relation to Dietary Fish Oil and Oxidative Stress in Elderly," *Free Radicals and Aging,* 1992; 411–18.

Oliveri, O. "Selenium Status, Fatty Acids, Vitamin A and E and Aging: The Nove Study," *American Journal of Clinical Nutrition,* 1994; 60:510–7.

Poeggeler, B., et al. "Melatonin, Hydroxyl Radical-Mediated Oxidative Damage and Aging," *Journal of Pineal Research,* 1993; 14:151–168.

Ward, J. "Free Radicals, Antioxidants and Preventive Geriatrics," *Australian Family Physician,* July 1994; 23(7):1297–1305.

Weindruch, R. "Calorie Restriction and Aging," *Scientific American,* January 1996; 46–52.

Sexual Vitality

Bernard, N. "Natural Progesterone: Is Estrogen the Wrong Hormone?" *Good Medicine,* Spring 1994; 11–13.

Carper, J. *The Food Pharmacy.* New York: Bantam, 1988.

Diokkno, A., et al. "Sexual Function in the Elderly," *Archives of Internal Medicine,* 1990; 150:197–200.

"High Cholesterol Diet Linked to Sex Problems," *Medical Tribune,* June 25; 1992:14.

Lieberman, S., Bruning, N. *The Real Vitamin & Mineral Book.* Garden City Park, NY: Avery Publishing Group, 1990.

Murray, M., Pizzorno, J. *Encyclopedia of Natural Medicine,* 2nd ed. Rocklin, CA: Prima Publishing, 1998.

Null, G. *Women's Encyclopedia of Natural Healing.* New York: Seven Stories Press, 1996.

O'Carroll, R., et al. "Testosterone Therapy for Low Sexual Interest and Erectile Dysfunction in Men: A Controlled Study," *British Journal of Psychiatry;* 145:146–51.

Pfieffer, E., et al. "Determinants of Sexual Behavior in Middle and Old Age," *Journal of the American Geriatrics Society,* XX(4):151–8.

Rowland, D. L. P. "Yohimbine, Erectile Capacity, and Sexual Response in Men," *Archives of Sexual Behavior,* 1997; 26(1):49–62.

White, J. R., et al. "Enhanced Sexual Behavior in Exercising Men," *Archives of Sexual Behavior,* 1990; 19(3):193–207.

Immune System Support

Abdallah, R. M., et al. "Astragalosides from Egyptian Astragalus Spinosus," *Val Pharmazie,* 1993; 48:452–454.

Balch, J. F., Balch, P. A. *Prescriptions for Nutritional Healing.* Garden City Park, NY: Avery Publishing Group, Inc., 1990.

Beyer, R. E. "An Analysis of the Role of Coenzyme Q in Free Radical Generation as an Antioxidant," *Biochemistry and Cell Biology,* 1991; 70:390–403.

Brandtzaeg, P. "Development and Basic Mechanisms of Human Gut Immunity," *Nutrition Reviews,* 56:S5–S18.

Calder, P. C. "Dietary Fatty Acids and the Immune Response," *Nutrition Reviews,* 1988; 56:S70–S83.

Cunningham-Rundles, S. "Analytical Methods for Evaluation of Immune Response in Nutrient Intervention," *Nutrition Reviews,* 1998; 56:S27–S37.

Failla, M. L., Hopkins, R. G. "Is Low Copper Status Immunosuppressive?" *Nutrition Reviews,* 56:S59–S64.

Folkers, K., et al. "The Activities of Coenzyme Q10 and Vitamin B_6 for Immune Response," *Biochemical and Biophysical Research Communications,* 1993; 193:88–92.

Gaby, A. R. "The Role of Coenzyme Q10 in Clinical Medicine: Part 1," *Alternative Medicine Review,* 1996; 1:11–17.

Grimble, R. F. "Effect of Antioxidative Vitamins on Immune Function with Clinical Applications," *International Journal for Vitamin & Nutrition Research,* 1997; 67:312–320.

Groff, J. L., Gropper, S. S., Hunt, S. M. *Advanced Nutrition and Human Metabolism,* 2nd ed. New York: West Publishing Co., 1995.

Hedge, H. R. "Nutrients as Modulators of Immune Function," *Canadian Medical Association Journal,* 1991; 145:1080–1081.

Keusch, G. T. "Nutrition and Immunity," *Nutrition Reviews,* 1998; 56:S3–S4.

Lai, Chiu-Nan. "The Active Factor in Wheat Sprout Extract Inhibiting the Metabolic Activation of Carcinogens in Vitro," *Nutrition and Cancer* 1(3):19–21. (In Kenton L., Kenton, S. *Raw Energy.* London: Century Publishing, 1985.)

Meydani, S. N., Beharka, A. A. "Recent Developments in Vitamin E and Immune Response," *Nutrition Reviews,* 1996; 56:S49–S58.

Murray, M., Pizzorno, J. *Encyclopedia of Natural Medicine,* 2nd ed. Rocklin, CA: Prima Publishing, 1998.

Schmidt, K. "Interaction of Antioxidative Micronutrients with Host Defense Mechanisms: A Critical Review," *International Journal for Vitamin & Nutrition Research,* 1997; 67:307–311.

Semba, R. D. "The Role of Vitamin A and Related Retinoids in Immune Function," *Nutrition Reviews,* 1998; 56:S38–S48.

Zhao, K. S., et al. "Enhancement of the Immune Response in Mice by Astragalus Membanaceu Extracts," *Immunopharmacology* 1990; 20:225–234.

Peak Memory and Mental Performance

Balch, J. F., Balch, P. A. *Prescription for Nutritional Healing.* Garden City Park, NY: Avery Publishing Group, Inc., 1990.

Grassel, E. "Effect of Ginkgo-Biloba Extract on Mental Performance: Double-Blind Study Using Computerized Measurement Conditions in Patients with Cerebral Insufficiency," *Fortschritte der Medizin,* February 20, 1992; 110(5):73–76.

Hutchinson, M. *Mega Brain Power.* New York: Hyperion, 1994.

Jaiswal, A. K., Bhattachatya, S. K. "Effects of Gestational Undernutrition, Stress, and Diazepam Treatment on Spatial Discrimination Learning and Retention in Young Rats," *Indian Journal of Experimental Biology,* April 1993; 31(4):353–359.

Kanowski, S., et al. "Proof of Efficacy of Ginkgo Biloba Special Extract EGb761 in Outpatients Suffering from Mild to Moderate Primary Dementia of the Alzheimer's Type or Multi-Infarct Dementia," *Phytomedicine,* 1997; 4(1):3–13.

La Rue, A., et al. "Nutritional Status and Cognitive Functioning in a Normally Aging Sample: A 6 Year Reassessment," *American Journal of Clinical Nutrition,* 65(1):20–29.

Lopez, I., et al. "Breakfast Omission and Cognitive Performance of Normal, Wasted, and Stunted Schoolchildren," *European Journal of Clinical Nutrition,* August 1993; 47(8):533–542.

Owens, B. D. "Blood Glucose and Human Memory," *Psychopharmacology,* 1993; 113(1):83–88.

Penland, J. G. "Dietary Boron, Brain Function, and Cognitive Performance," *Environmental Health Perspectives,* November 1994; 102(7):65–72.

Pollitt, E. "Does Breakfast Make a Difference in School?" *Journal of the American Dietetic Association,* October 1995; 95(10):1134–1139.

Pollitt, E., et al. "Three-Month Nutritional Supplementation in Indonesian Infants and Toddlers Benefits Memory Function 8 Years Later," *American Journal of Clinical Nutrition,* December 1997; 66(6):1357–1363.

Richter, L. M., et al. "Cognitive and Behavioral Effects of a School Breakfast," *South African Medical Journal,* January 1997; 87(1):93–100.

Wecker, L. "Neurochemical Effects of Choline Supplementation," *Canadian Journal of Physiology and Pharmacology,* March 1986; 64(3):329–333.

Wong, K. L., et al. "Dietary cis-Fatty Acids That Increase Protein F1 Phosphorylation Enhance Spatial Memory," *Brain Research,* December 1989; 505(2):302–305.

Wood, J. L., Allison, R. G. "Effects of Consumption of Choline and Lecithin on Neurological and Cardiovascular Systems," *Federation Proceedings,* December 1982; 41(14):3015–3021.

Zeisel, S. H. "Choline: An Important Nutrient in Brain Development, Liver Function, and Carcinogenesis," *Journal of the American College of Nutrition,* October 1992; 11(5):473–481.

Zeisel, S. H. "Choline Was Essential for Brain Development and Function," *Advances in Pediatrics,* 1997; 44:263–295.

Enhancing Job Performance

Bahrke, M. S., and Morgan, W. P. "Evaluation of Erogenic Properties of Ginseng," *Sports Medicine,* 1994; 18(4):229–248.

Benton, D., and Cook, R. "The Impact of Selenium Supplementation on Mood," *Biological Psychiatry,* June 1991; 29(11):1092–8.

Clark, N. "The Power of Protein," *The Physician and Sports Medicine,* April 1996; 24(4):11–12.

Ellis, F. R., and Nassar, S. "A Pilot Study of Vitamin B_{12} in the Treatment of Tiredness," *British Journal of Nutrition,* 1973; 30:277–83.

Kenton, L., and Kenton, S. *Raw Energy.* London: Century Publishing, 1985.

Pizzorno, J. E., and Murray, M. T. *The Textbook of Natural Medicine.* Seattle, WA: Bastyr University Publications, 1992.

"Specific Nutrients Aid in High-Performance Activity," *Nutrition Week,* June 10, 1994; 7.

Exercise and Sports Endurance

Anderson, R. A., et al. "Chromium and Its Role in Lean Body Mass and Weight Reduction," *The Nutrition Report,* June 1993; 11(6):41–46.

Bahrke, M. S., and Morgan, W. P. "Evaluation of the Erogenic Properties of Ginseng," *Sports Medicine,* 1994; 18(4):229–248.

Calbom, C. "Drink Your Vegetables," *Women's Sports and Fitness,* September 1992.

Clark, N. "The Power of Protein," *The Physician and Sports Medicine,* April 1996; 24(4):11–12.

Giuliani, A., and Cestaro, B. "Exercise, Free Radical Generation and Vitamins," *European Journal of Cancer Prevention,* 1997; 6(1):S55–S67.

Kanter, M. M. "Free Radicals, Exercise, and Antioxidant Supplementation," *International Journal of Sports Nutrition,* 1994; 4:205–220.

Kleiner, S. "Healthy Muscle Gains," *The Physician and Sports Medicine,* April 1995; 23(4):21–22.

Kleiner, S. "The Lowdown on Carbo Loading," *The Physician and Sports Medicine,* August 1995; 23(8):19–20.

Rhein, R. "Antioxidants Let Weekend Athletes Avoid Soreness," *Family Practice News,* August 1, 1996; 32.

Simon-Schnass, I. M. "Nutrition and High Altitude," *Journal of Nutrition* 1992; 122:778–781.

Swart, I., et al. "The Effect of L-Carnitine Supplementation on Plasma Carnitine Levels and Various Performance Parameters of Male Marathon Athletes," *Nutrition Research,* 1997; 17(3):405–414.

"The Surgeon General's Report: A Primary Resource for Exercise Advocates," *The Physician and Sports Medicine,* April 1997; 25(4):122–131.

Vasankari, T. J., et al. "Increased Serum and Low-Density-Lipoprotein Antioxidant Potential After Antioxidant Supplementation in Endurance Athletes," *American Journal of Clinical Nutrition,* 1997; 65:1052–1056.

Weight Loss

Anderson, R. A., et al. "Chromium and Its Role in Lean Body Mass and Weight Reduction," *The Nutrition Report,* June 1993; 11(6):41–46.

"Appetite and High Fat Foods," *Nutrition Week,* March 28, 1997; 27(12):7.

"Aspartame and Dieting," *Nutrition Week,* June 13, 1997; 27(23):7/*International Journal of Obesity,* January 1997; 21(1):37–42.

Evans, G. W., Pouchnik D. J. "Composition and Biological Activity of Chromium-Pyridine Carbosylate Complexes," *Journal of Inorganic Biochemistry,* 1993; 49: 177–187.

McCarty, M. F. "The Prophylactic and Therapeutic Potential of Chromium Picolinate and Diabetes Mellitus, Hyperlipidemia, Anabolism and Weight Reduction," *Journal of Advancement in Medicine,* spring 1993; 6(1):47–52.

"Pantothenic Acid and Weight Loss," *The Nutrition Report,* September 1995; 61.

Rossner, S., et al. "Weight Reduction with Dietary Fibre Supplements: Results of Two Double-Blind Studies," *Acta Medica Scandinavica,* 1987; 22:83–88.

Juicing for Babies and Children

Boschert, S. "How Well Are You Counseling Mothers?" *Family Practice News,* September 1, 1995; 121.

"Child Obesity Rising, Says Public Voice Conference," *Nutrition Week,* June 23, 1995; 25(24):3.

Clausen, S. W. "Carotenes and Resistance to Infection," *Transactions of the American Pediatric Society,* 1931; 43:27–30.

Dennison, B. A. "Fruit Juice Consumption by Infants and Children: A Review," *Journal of the American College of Nutrition,* 1996; 15(5):4S–11S.

Dewey, K. G., et al. "Growth of Breast Fed and Formula Fed Infants From 0 to 18 Months: The DARLING Study," *Pediatrics,* June 1992; 89(6):1035–1041.

Keane, M. B. *Juicing for Good Health.* New York: Pocket Books, 1992.

Krebs-Smith, S. M., et al. "Fruit and Vegetable Intake of Children and Adolescents in the United States," *Archives of Pediatrics and Adolescent Medicine,* January 1996; 150:81–86.

"Over 7,000 Aspartame Complaints Since '81, FDA Says; Controversy Remains," *Nutrition Week,* May 26, 1995; 25(20):1–2.

Raloff, J. "Microwaving Can Lower Breast Milk Benefits," *Science News,* April 25, 1992; 141:261.

Sullivan, S. A., Birch, L. L. "Infant Dietary Experience and Acceptance of Solid Foods," *Pediatrics,* February 1994; 93(2):271–277.

"The Use of Whole Cow's Milk in Infancy: Committee on Nutrition," *Pediatrics,* June 1992; 89(6):1105–1107.

Wagner, C. L., et al. "Special Properties of Human Milk," *Clinical Pediatrics,* June 1996; 283–293.

Healthy Pregnancy

Berger, H. *Vitamins and Minerals in Pregnancy and Lactation.* New York: Raven Press, 1998.

Carper, J. *Food—Your Miracle Medicine.* New York: HarperCollins Publishers, 1993.

Czeizel, A. E., Hirschberg, J. "Orofacial Clefts in Hungary, Epidemiological and Genetic Data, Primary Prevention," *Folia Phoniatrica et Logopedica,* 1997; 49:111–116.

Erasmus, U. "Infants and Oils," *Fats That Heal; Fats That Kill.* Burnaby, BC, Canada: Alive Books, 1993.

Guthrie, H. A. *Human Nutrition.* St. Louis, MO: Mosby Publishing, 1995.

Jacobson, J. L., et al. "Effects of in Utero Exposure to Polychlorinated Biphenyls and Related Contaminants on Cognitive Functioning in Young Children," *Journal of Pediatrics,* January 1990; 116(1):38–45.

Keane, M. B. *Juicing for Good Health.* New York: Pocket Books, 1992.

Lieberman, S., Bruning, N. "Vitamin B_6 (Pyridoxine)," *The Real Vitamin Mineral Book.* Garden City Park, NY: Avery Publishing Group, Inc., 1990.

Menard, M. K. "Vitamin and Mineral Supplementation Prior to and During Pregnancy," *Obstetrics and Gynecology Clinics of North America,* September 1997; 24:479–8.

Murray, M. T. *The Healing Power of Foods.* Rocklin, CA: Prima Publishing, 1993.

Murray, M. T. "Essential Fatty Acid Supplementation," *Encyclopedia of Nutritional Supplements.* Rocklin, CA: Prima Publishing, 1996.

Preston, M. S., et al. "Maternal Consumption of Cured Meats and Vitamins in Relation to Pediatric Brain Tumors," *Cancer Epidemiology, Biomarkers and Prevention,* August 1996; 5:599–605.

Scholl, T. O., Hediger, M. L. "Use of Multivitamin/Mineral Prenatal Supplements: Influence on the Outcome of Pregnancy," *American Journal of Epidemiology,* July 1997; 146:134–141.

Shaw, G. M., et al. "Low Birth Weight, Preterm Delivery, and Periconception Vitamin Use," *Journal of Pediatrics,* June 1997; 130:1013–1014.

Swinney, B. *Eating Expectantly: The Essential Guide and Cookbook for Pregnancy.* Colorado Springs, CO: Fall Rivers Press, 1993.

Zeisel, S. H. "Choline: Essential for Brain Development and Function," *Advances in Pediatrics,* 1997; 44:263–295.

Healthy Breast-feeding

"Breast Feeding Moms: Shun Alcohol, but Eat Garlic?" *Human Sexuality,* January 1992; 26(1):16.

Keane, M. B. *Juicing for Good Health.* New York: Pocket Books, 1992.

Lieberman, S., Bruning, N. *The Real Vitamin & Mineral Book.* Garden City Park, NY: Avery Publishing Group, 1990.

Richardson, A. "Diabetes and Schizophrenia: Genes of Zinc Deficiency?" *The Lancet,* November 7, 1992; 340:1160.

Juicy Tips for Pets

Bowers, T. L. "Nutrition and Immunity Part 2: The Role of Selected Micronutrients and Clinical Significance," *Veterinary Clinical Nutrition,* 1997; 4(3):96–101.

Goldstein, B., Goldstein, S. *Love of Animals,* April, vol. 3(4); May, vol. 3(5), 1998.

Organically Grown

Benbrook, Charles. "How to Avoid Pesticides," *Nutrition Action,* June 1997.

Cimmons, M., et al. "U.S. OKs Irradiation to Purify Meat," *Los Angeles Times,* December 3, 1997; A4.

Crinnion, Walter J. "Better Living with Organic Foods," *Delicious,* April 1995.

Diehl, J. F. "Irradiate Food," *Science,* 1973; 180(82):214–215.

Gussow, Jane D. "But Is It More Nutritious?" *Eating Well,* May/June 1997.

Meeker-Lowry, S., et al. "Nuclear Lunch: The Dangers and Unknowns of Food Irradiation," *Food and Water Journal,* fall/winter 1997; 17–21.

"Organic Tomatoes, Vitamin C and Calcium," *Nutrition Week,* June 19, 1998; 28(24):7/*Hort/Science,* April 1998; 33(2):255–257.

Rhea, W. J., Liang, H.-C. "Effects of Pesticides on the Immune System," *Journal of Nutritional Medicine,* 1991; 2:399–410.

Weil, Andrew, M.D. *8 Weeks to Optimum Health.* New York: Alfred A. Knopf, 1997, 167.

Weisenburger, D. D. "Human Health Effects of Agrichemical Use," *Human Pathology,* June 1993; 24(6):571–576.

Index

beta carotene, 6
  in cantaloupe, 66
  in fruits, 35
  and longevity, 72
  as oxygen quencher, 124
bile, 159, 165
bioelectrical energy, 22
bioflavonoids
  capillary-strengthening properties of, 81
  in lemons, 37
  for skin health, 92
biotechnology, 181
biotin, 85
bladder wrack (*Fucus vesiculous*), 82, 134
blood pressure, and magnesium, 58
blood sugar level, maintenance of, 134
body consciousness, 195
body-food-health connection, 1, 190
bone support
  Bone Power Plus, 57
  See also calcium
boron, for mental performance, 118
brainpower, support for, 116–122
bread, 177
breast-feeding, 136–137
  health maintenance during, 150–152
breast milk, heating of, 137
bromelain, 95. *See also* pineapple juice
Brown, Lester, 181
Brunzi, 195–197
Brunzi's Best, 196
Brussels sprouts, in Jack and the Bean, 31–32
bulking agents, for cleansing programs, 161
Butler, Jade, 179

cabbage juice
  for immune system support, 112, 115
  for skin health, 93
  Triple C, 20
caffeine, avoiding, 101, 121
calcium
  from Beautiful Bone Solution, 25
  for children, 143
  for facial/cranial bone maintenance, 92
  for lactating women, 152
  for pregnant women, 148
  Sweet Calcium Cocktail, 24
  Sweet Dreams Nightcap, 29–30
calories
  for lactating women, 150
  reducing, to look younger, 72
cancer
  and aspartame, 48
  beta carotene, vitamin C, and provitamin
    A, effects on, 35

and phytochemicals, 10
  skin, prevention of, 91
  spinach juice for, 21
  strawberries for, 64
  testicular, 191–192
candidiasis, 2
  fruit juices, avoidance of, 35
canola oil, 76
cantaloupes and cantaloupe juice
  Cantaloupe Sorbet, 66
  Strawberry-Cantaloupe Cocktail, 38
carbohydrate loading, 129–130
carbohydrates, 8
carbohydrates, complex, 174
  for brainpower, 120
  for cellulite prevention, 80
  for muscle support, 126–127
  for pregnant women, 146
carbohydrates, simple
  avoidance of, and cellulite prevention,
    80
  and immune system functioning, 112
carotenes
  for children, 142
  for immune system support, 113
  for longevity, 72, 105
  for pets, 156
  for skin health, 77, 91
carotenoids, 73
  in cantaloupe, 38
  in oranges, 63
  in papaya, 60
carrot greens, removing, 7
carrot juice
  for children, 140
  for hair loss, 193–194
  for looking younger, 74
  for pets, 154–155
  for sexual vitality, 109
  for skin health, 93
  Sweet Dreams Nightcap, 29–30
  Weight Loss Buddy, 29
Carrot Salad, 169
cats, juicing for, 153–158
cauliflower, in Memory Mender, 27–28
celery juice
  for looking younger, 74
  for pets, 154–155
  sodium in, 155
  storage of, 16
  Sweet Dreams Nightcap, 29–30
  Waldorf Twist, 16
cellulite prevention/correction, 79–83
  Anticellulite Massage Oil Formula, 82
  Cellulite Corrector, 82

malaria, 190
male pattern baldness, 192–194
mango juice, in Mango Mania, 57–58
Marangoni, Carol, 195–197
massage, for cellulite prevention, 81
Massage, Hair-Grow Scalp, 87
Mayville, Bill, Sr., and Patricia, 194–195
meal replacements. *See* smoothies
meat consumption, 178, 192–193
medical establishment, 200
  blind faith in, 193
Mega Brain Power (Hutchinson), 119
melatonin, 73
  for longevity, 105
melons and melon juices
  Cantaloupe Sorbet, 66
  Minty Melon Cooler, 45
  Minty Melon Refresher, 53
  for pets, 155
  Strawberry-Cantaloupe Cocktail, 38
  Watermelon Refresher, 40
memory support, 116–119
  Memory Mender, 27–28
mental performance support, 116–119
milk
  for babies, 137, 138
  recommended intake of, 178
milk thistle (silymarin), 170
minerals, 9–10
mint
  After-Dinner Mint, 43
  Lemon-Mint Sorbet, 66–67
  Mint Medley, 23
  Minty Melon Cooler, 45
  Minty Melon Refresher, 53
moods, and selenium intake, 102
Morning Energizer, 16
morning sickness, Snappy Ginger for, 38
Morning Sunrise, 39–40
Mt. Shasta Herb and health, skin cleansing
    program from, 172
muscle support, Muscle Power Plus, 56

nail health, 84–87
  Beautiful Skin, Hair, and Nails Cocktail, 24
  Spicy Coconut Delight, 61
National Cancer Institute, 10, 35
Nature's Best Electrolyte Replacer, 46, 130
nausea, Snappy Ginger for, 38
nerves, calming of, 16
nettles root, for sexual vitality, 109
nettles tea, 168
neurotransmitters, 118
nicotine, avoiding, 101, 104, 108, 121
NutraSweet, 133

nutrient deficiencies, and hair and nail
    health, 84
nutrients
  cooking and freezing, effects on, 6
  time effects on, 8
nuts, recommended intake of, 178

oils
  rancid, avoidance of, 76
  recommended intake of, 179
Oldfield, Harry, 175
olive oil, 76
Optimum Health Institute (OHI), 91, 160
orange juice
  benefits of, 23
  creamsicles with, 67
  and grapefruit, for children, 140
  Grapefruit-Orange Spritzer, 52
  Morning Express, 20
  Morning Sunrise, 39–40
  Orange-Apple Cooler, 51–52
  Orange Sorbet, 63–64
  Orange Velvet, 23
  Rise 'n' Shake, 55
organic farming, 180–182
  information on, 201
organic produce, 6, 7, 13, 180–183, 193–194
  consumption during pregnancy, 146
  suppliers of, 201

panax ginseng
  for energy, 102
  for physical and mental performance
    improvement, 122
pancreas support, Jack and the Bean for,
    31–32
pantothenic acid
  for fat metabolism, 133
  for stress relief, 121
papaya
  for exfoliating, 91
  Papaya Peeler, 95
  Tropical Treat, 60
parasites, 164
parsley, 17, 134
  Beautiful Bone Solution, 25
  Champ smoothie, 56
  Parsley Pep, 26
  Sweet Dreams Nightcap, 29–30
  Weight-Loss Express, 28–29
  for youthful appearance, 74
parsnip juice
  Beautiful Skin, Hair, and Nails Cocktail, 24
  and carrots, for skin health, 93
pasta, 177

THE JUICE LADY™ PRO JUICER

The Juicer That's Changing America's Health Habits

IT'S SO EASY; MY JUICER HAS . . .

▷ Large feed tube and powerful .50-hp motor for faster juicing—skins, stems, rinds, and all.
▷ Dishwasher-safe, snap-apart components; cleanup and assembly are a snap.
▷ Oversized, freestanding pulp receptacle for nonstop juicing.
▷ Stainless steel parts.

SO GOOD FOR YOU!

Razor-sharp stainless steel blade basket gets more juice from your produce. A delicious way to consume 3 to 5 servings of vegetables and 2 to 4 servings of fruit each day, as recommended by the USDA Food Guide Pyramid.

COMPREHENSIVE NUTRITIONAL AND OPERATIONAL INFORMATION

You'll receive my personal Juice Lady™ Recipe and Menu Planner. Instruction Manual—covers every aspect of using and caring for the Pro Juicer.

THE JUICE LADY™ ENERGY FORMULA

Turn Your Juice into Super Juice!

COMPLETE WHOLE FOOD NUTRITION
▷ with Vitamins, Minerals, Energizing Botanicals, Active Cultures, and Isoflavones ▷ Delicious French Vanilla ▷ No Sugar Added

MY *Juice Lady™ Energy Formula* is a powder supplement designed to mix easily with fresh fruit and vegetable juices. It offers an abundance of cold-processed plant foods and compounds that have their enzymes and nutrients intact. When combined with fresh juice, it becomes the source of optimum nourishment for the body. If you feel fatigued, work out regularly, or want to lose weight, my formula will give your juice a super boost of nutrients that will help you reach your goals. In most cases, this energy drink can become a complete meal replacement or snack, which will facilitate weight loss and super-boost your energy levels. It will turn your juice into "super juice."

To order, or for more information, call 1-800-233-9054.
Or write to me at the following address:
Juice Lady ▶ P.O. Box 380 ▶ Mt. Prospect, IL 60056